# THE GREAT AMERICAN DETOX DIET

## ALEX JAMIESON

RODALE

Printed in the United States of America
Rodale Inc. makes every effort to use acid-free ⊛, recycled paper ♻.

The paragraph on pages 67 and 68 is excerpted from *Breaking the Food Seduction*
by Neal Barnard, MD. Copyright © 2003 by the author
and reprinted by permission of St. Martin's Press, LLC.

Cover photograph by Juliet Piddington
Cover concept and design by Simon Daley
Interior design by Patricia Field

**Library of Congress Cataloging-in-Publication Data**

Jamieson, Alex.
    The great American detox diet : 8 weeks to weight loss and well-being / Alex
Jamieson.
        p.    cm.
    Includes index.
    ISBN-13 978–1–59486–231–1 hardcover
    ISBN-10 1–59486–231–1 hardcover
    ISBN-13 978–1–59486–484–1 paperback
    ISBN-10 1–59486–484–5 paperback
    1. Detoxification (Health)   2. Food habits—United States.   3. Nutrition.
4. Weight loss.   5. Spurlock, Morgan, date.   I. Title.
RA784.5.J35   2005
613.2'5—dc22                                                    2005005984

**Distributed to the trade by Holtzbrinck Publishers**

2   4   6   8   10   9   7   5   3   1   hardcover
2   4   6   8   10   9   7   5   3   1   paperback

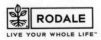

We inspire and enable people to improve their lives and the world around them

For more of our products visit **rodalestore.com** or call 800-848-4735

*To Mom, who taught me how to grow nature's bounty and use it for good food and health.*

*To Dad, who taught me the value of humor and working hard to save even one starfish.*

*To my Valentine, who inspires me every day to work and go after my dreams.*

*Thank you all for believing in me. I love you all.*

"PROBLEMS CANNOT BE SOLVED AT THE SAME LEVEL OF
AWARENESS THAT CREATED THEM."

—ALBERT EINSTEIN

# Contents

# *Super Size Me:* The Aftermath

It was Thanksgiving 2002 when I got the brilliant idea to send my body into a fast-food frenzy by eating McDonald's food for 30 days straight and make a movie about it. I was watching the news, when a story came on about two overweight, sick girls who were suing the House of Ronald for misleading them with their marketing claim that their food was healthful. At first, I thought these girls were crazy, but the more I learned about how fast-food restaurants (and the Golden Arches in particular) target kids in their marketing, how they manufacture their food, and how they hide the true nutritional content of that food from their customers, I thought, "There's definitely the basis here for an argument."

But back to that Thanksgiving day. While I sat on the couch, a spokesman for Ronny boy came on the TV and said that you can't link their food to these girls being sick; you can't link their food to these girls being obese. Their food "is healthy, it's nutritious . . . it's good for you!"

That's when the lightbulb went off and I got the idea for *Super Size Me.* I then turned to the person sitting next to me to share my epiphany. That person was my beautiful, longtime vegan girlfriend, Alex Jamieson. Needless to say, Alex did not share my enthusiasm for the project.

From the beginning, Alex was the one consistent voice warning me that this was a truly bad idea and would be profoundly bad for my health. I excel at being the stubborn boyfriend, so I didn't listen to her. Instead, I dove into this gastrointestinal form of hari-kari with the vigor and passion of a child who has been let loose in a candy store—or a McDonald's.

I did have to make one promise to Alex prior to filming. The deal was that she would agree to let me make this film, to eat this awful food that she knew to be exceptionally bad for me (even worse than I or my doctors imagined) on one condition: After the 30 days were over, my diet was hers. This was nonnegotiable.

The changes my body went through during the month were inconceivable. While eating all that fast food, I experienced three different health problems that, not coincidentally, we treat routinely in this country with massive amounts of prescription medication:

- I was massively depressed. I would eat the food and feel great for about an hour, but then I would hit the wall and be angry and moody and sad and depressed. I was a roller coaster emotionally for the entire month and showed many of the signs of clinical depression and bipolarity that we medicate the masses for every day with drugs like Prozac.

- I experienced sexual dysfunction, a problem that millions of men across America take Viagra to fix. (Alex, by the way, shared this tidbit about my health with millions of people worldwide in the film.)

- And last, my mind was all over the place. I couldn't focus. I couldn't pay attention. I had all the telltale signs of Attention Deficit Disorder (ADD), a mental condition that millions of kids in this country are diagnosed with and medicated for annually.

On top of this, my liver became filled with fat, my cholesterol skyrocketed, my blood pressure went through the roof, and I was now carrying around a gut with 24.5 additional pounds of McLove stuffed into it. And this, mind you, was after just 1 month.

When my 30-day commitment ended, I immediately began Alex's "Detox Diet," a diet she specifically designed to help my body deal with the problems it was facing and overcome the punishment it had been put through. At first, I went through massive withdrawal, much like what a drug addict or alcoholic experiences when detoxifying. My body craved the fat, sugar, sodium, and caffeine it had been overdosing on for the past month. I had massive headaches, I experienced periods of sweating and the shakes, and my body ached as though someone had beaten me with a large club. But over the next few days and weeks, I began to feel my focus sharpening, my energy levels increasing, my libido returning, and my personality coming back to what it was before I became a "hopped-up" junk-food junkie.

Many tried to discredit *Super Size Me* by saying that it was no surprise I became ill, when you take into account the number of calories I was eating; others say that the film and my experiment are quite representative of what can happen to your body from years of eating a diet high in fat, sugar, and processed food. In fact, in January 2005, the highly respected medical journal *The Lancet* released the results of a 15-year study that monitored more than 3,000 people who ate fast food only twice a week. Over this period, the subjects not only gained weight, but many of them also developed serious conditions, like insulin resistance, which is a precursor to diabetes.

The things my body went through while I was eating all that fast food should stand as a reminder of what types of food we should be avoiding as often as possible. I am thankful to have had someone like Alex there for me as I began my detox and recovery and rediscovered what real food tastes like.

I truly believe that she helped save my life by nursing my body back to health with care, kindness, and delicious food.

If you are persistent and follow the examples and suggestions Alex makes in this book, I believe you'll emerge from the other side of your 8-week detox just as I did: feeling energized, focused, healthy, alive, and, most important, quite thankful that Alex was there to help.

Happy eating!

—MORGAN SPURLOCK, creator and
director of *Super Size Me:
A Film of Epic Portions*

# The Benefits of Preventive Eating

"*The Great American Detox Diet* is a truly groundbreaking primer on the benefits of what I call preventive eating. As a doctor, I truly see that 'an ounce of prevention is worth a pound of cure,' especially when it comes to our diets."

—LISA GANJHU, DO

**I was introduced to Alex Jamieson** while at the Sundance Film Festival. Both of us were there because we were involved in the remarkable film *Super Size Me,* the eye-opening documentary by Morgan Spurlock about fast food. Alex and I talked about what she does and how she integrates nutrition and cooking. I was impressed with her approach to nutrition and healthy living. I practice in a similar way. I believe our health starts with the fuels we give our bodies. As a gastroenterologist, I know that how and what we feed ourselves either enhances or destroys our digestive health.

I was honored when Alex asked me to write a foreword to her book. I read the book while it was still a manuscript, and I couldn't put it down. I learned so much about healthy eating, and I loved Alex's recipes so much that I began to apply her detox plan to myself and my patients. This book is a wonderful resource for those who want to make real changes in their lives, starting with the basics.

In a voice that is supportive and intelligent and that adds a sense of fun and playfulness to our thinking about food, Alex outlines how and why our diets have become so nutrient-poor and how easy it is to get them back on track. She has a keen understanding of why substances like sugar and caffeine are so addictive, and she offers tips and recipes that will make giving up these harmful things easy and enjoyable.

Alex talks about nutrition in easy-to-understand language and gently reminds us that no two human beings are the same and so no one diet works for all of us. In fact, she takes the brilliant step of saying that we shouldn't even think about dieting. Instead, we should think about detoxing our bodies by replacing unhealthy foods with wholesome food fuels.

Alex also teaches us about alternative sources of nutrition. I now have a better understanding of the broad range of diets my patients follow (I used to think quinoa was a bird and millet was a haircut). Alex has created recipes that are flavorful and delicious. I particularly like her healthy alternatives to "old favorites."

Too many modern health problems can be traced back to a poor diet. Many Americans are considered overfed, yet they are undernourished. Diseases such as diabetes and obesity and their associated complications are related to an imbalance of consumption and metabolism. Simply said, people are eating too much but are not burning off the extra calories. Portion control is an important part of healthy eating. It also matters what quality of food we put into our mouths.

My medical training in nutrition was only for the very ill—those patients who literally could not feed themselves. Like most doctors today, I did not get any formal training in preventative nutrition, and this, I now realize, is a serious shortcoming of our medical education system. Physicians must talk to their patients about their diets and encourage them to select healthy foods. In doing so, they may prevent diseases. I have made talking about diets a major part of my evaluation of all my patients.

As Alex Jamieson so eloquently shows us in this book, healthy eating is really quite simple. It is all about quality and portion size. Make the right choices and eat in moderation, and you will enjoy excellent health. That is the simple yet profound message of *The Great American Detox Diet.*

—Lisa Ganjhu, D.O., attending physician in the division of gastroenterology and liver diseases at St. Luke's-Roosevelt Hospital Center, and assistant clinical professor of medicine at Columbia University College of Physicians and Surgeons, both in New York City

## PART ONE

# DON'T DIET—
# DETOX!

# My Own Detox Experience

I was raised in a bohemian, socially conscious family in Oregon in the '70s and '80s, and the overall memory I have of that time is the recollection of feeling exquisitely well, fit, and happy as a child. I don't ever remember lacking the energy to do anything, be it doing chores, participating in sports, tackling schoolwork, or just giving myself up to rowdy, exuberant play. I never, ever gave my weight a thought or contemplated whether what I put into my mouth was good for me or not.

My father was a high school teacher who also coached swimming and soccer. My mother (who had my older brother when she was just 21) was voraciously artistic. Even while caring for my brother (and 6 years after his arrival, me), she studied art, architecture, landscaping, and any other form of visual art that fired her incredible imagination. One of her great passions was our organic garden. I call it a garden, but it was really a minifarm, where we grew herbs, greens, fruit, berries, beans, flowers, tomatoes, and blackberries (though we hardly *grew* the blackberries—we were simply fighting a never-ending war of pruning and hacking back wildly hearty vines in a futile attempt to rediscover a garden path). Sometimes I think Brendan and I were born just so Mom and Dad would have a crew on hand to help prune, weed, and haul firewood. Every weekend, rain or shine, the entire family would be outside working together, growing our own food and creating our own piece of paradise in the soggy Oregon earth. By the time I was 5 years old, my mother was hosting a weekly radio show called "Eve's Organic Garden," and she even became something of a local celebrity. My father thought this was great, because he was a big believer in doing your part as a citizen and giving back to your community. I guess that's where my roots started: in the fertile soil of my down-to-earth family, who believed passionately in idealism, civic duty, hard work, and homegrown food.

My parents were both great cooks, and because we were living on a teacher's salary, their creativity in the kitchen was a real blessing. My father grew up in Louisiana, so he had a real love for spicy, Cajun-inspired foods. My mother's early years were spent in Texas, where she fell in love with southwestern spices and ingredients. She later traveled to Peru, Spain, and Asia, and all of those influences were found at our table. My parents weren't the only ones in their circle who were interested in raising their own food. They had friends who kept bees, so we had fresh, organic honey. Other friends kept chickens and shared their organic eggs with us. Still others, who grew berries and fruits that we didn't raise, swapped them for our blackberries and other produce. At least a couple of times a year, the whole family would pile into the car and drive to a you-pick farm, where we'd spend the day harvesting whatever was in season: hazelnuts, apples, or cherries. We'd pick an insane amount of whatever was fresh and eat all of it; then we'd set our sights on the next natural treat that the calendar brought.

Breakfast in my childhood home was usually whole grain cereal, fruit, and milk. We weren't allowed to have sugary store-bought cereals (too expensive!), so the most exciting thing we ever bought from the cereal aisle was Cheerios. Our mom taught us while young how to prepare our own lunches, so I'd usually make myself a peanut-butter-and-banana sandwich and take that to school with at least one piece of fruit. I was allowed to buy a hot lunch in the cafeteria 1 day a week, and I always scanned the lunch calendar for one of my favorite (and forbidden at home) treats. Friday was chocolate-milk day, so I usually chose hot lunch on Friday. We always ate dinner together as a family, and I remember that we ate lots of delicious casseroles, stews, and interesting combinations of whatever local fresh produce was available.

Because we weren't raised to be snackers, and we rarely had any junk food in our house (there was no room in our food budget for any of this), my parents made treats and lovely desserts for us from the fruits we grew in our own garden. Dad made killer blackberry cobblers and homemade vanilla ice cream. Mom preserved fresh raspberry jam and baked rhubarb crisp in the spring. She even made goodies out of carob, which, unlike chocolate, is caffeine-free. But even back then, though I hadn't yet had my fill of candy bars, my native "chocoholic" radar detected carob as being something of an imposter. It wasn't until years later that I discovered the great joys of carob and began to use it in delicious and satisfying recipes myself.

Despite my parents' best efforts to provide a wholesome diet, I was always trying to find ways to get my hands on sugary treats to satisfy my huge sweet tooth. I got a monthly allowance of $5, and as soon as I had that money in hand, I'd head straight to the candy store. But $5 didn't buy me enough sugar to get me through the month, so my friend Anna and I would scrounge up change or find bottles and cans that we could return for a nickel deposit on each. When we had a handful of change, we'd go right back to the candy store.

Every Christmas, my grandparents would send us a huge tin of cookies, which my parents would dole out to us at the excruciating rate of one cookie per meal. Of course, given my sweet tooth, I would steal into the kitchen on many nights, break into the stash, and help myself to a few extra cookies.

When I look back on it now, I see that my parents gave me and my brother a great gift in that they fed us a diet that was built around fresh whole foods that were grown locally (and often organically), and they limited our intake of refined sugar (I do remember the occasional Dr. Pepper in the summertime) in a way that felt, well, normal. But this being America, and I having been born with an outrageous sweet tooth, my diet was not destined to stay as healthy and well balanced for long. The way I ate changed radically when I got my first job at a place called Muffin Break.

I was 14 years old at the time, and I was desperate to have some discretionary spending money so I could be like my friends and shop at the mall, eat at fast-food restaurants, and buy as much candy and soda as I wanted. I started as a lowly dishwasher, but I had access to all the yummy treats and leftovers I could stomach. I especially loved their sugary blueberry muffins, which were as rich as wedding cake and not at all the healthful breakfast food they were advertised to be. Once I got my fill of the muffins, I'd guzzle soda and munch on cookies for the rest of the day. By the time I got home for dinner, I was too full to look at the wholesome, delicious meals my mother always had ready for us.

Were I asked now to pinpoint when my addiction to sugar started, I guess I would have to credit it to my time at Muffin Break. I was so habituated to junk food (anything with sugar, fat, or salt as a primary ingredient) that when I got to high school, I worked at a succession of low-paying jobs (in a dog-grooming parlor, at a video rental store, in a Mexican restaurant as the hostess) that brought me tiny paychecks that were just big enough to keep the tank of my light-blue '66 Volvo full of gas and my stomach full of Big Macs, Super Big Gulps, and 100 Grand chocolate bars. Probably because I had had a great whole foods diet as a child, and probably because I was the beneficiary of a lucky roll of the genetic dice, I didn't gain an ounce during high school, and I continued to shoot straight up until I reached my current height of 5 feet 10 inches at the age of 17.

Going off to college didn't make me any smarter about my diet. I spent my food credits in the dorm complex cafeteria on grade D meats, sugared cereals, giant cookies, pretzels, pizzas, burgers, fries, and sodas. It's amazing that I was able to study with all that sugar and caffeine running through my blood. Still, my high metabolism kept pace. I could throw down huge quantities of barbequed-chicken pizza dipped in ranch dressing, and I still wouldn't feel any snugness in my jeans the next day.

I spent the first few years after college traveling around, trying different cities, jobs, and lifestyles. I went to San Francisco and worked in advertising; then I moved north to Lake Tahoe and lived as a snow bunny/conference planner; from there, I headed to New York City, where I worked as a legal assistant at a high-powered entertainment law firm, and where my lousy diet finally caught up with me. The only constant in my life during those years was my diet, which was built around my love for coffee, cheese, chocolate, and *anything* with sugar in it. Wherever I was living, whatever work I was doing, I always practiced the weekly ritual of baking double-chocolate-chip cookies. I would give half of each batch to friends and coworkers and eat the rest myself.

It was a desk job that finally did me in, or at least slowed me down enough so that my body finally spoke up and cried uncle. I began to feel bad in ways I had never experienced before. For the first time in my life, I started to gain weight and I felt depressed. Energy seemed to be draining from my body like fuel dripping out of a gas tank with a hole in it. I had terrible migraine headaches for the first time in my life, too. My response to these symptoms was to drink more coffee, eat more chocolate, and continue to fill up on carbohydrates, in a blind attempt to restart my engine. But this way of eating—even for quick, nutrient-poor energy—failed me. I began to sense that something was seriously wrong. Over Christmas 1999, I was laid up while I recovered from knee surgery (brought on by one too many snowboarding spills), and my debilitating, mysterious symptoms got worse and worse. I took powerful antibiotics after my surgery, and those seemed to make me crave even more coffee, sugar, and pizza. While I ate more and more, I was also trapped at my desk every day in a windowless, airless office where the fluorescent lights hummed like a power plant. I was terribly bored at that job (my boss, who was lovely, needed me only to redraft his letters and briefs or answer the phone, and I would sit idle for long stretches, waiting for him to deliver work to me), so I began listening to a health-related program on talk radio hosted by Gary Null.

The topics covered on the show opened my eyes to a world of alternative diets and health and the connection of both to environmental issues. I was particularly struck by the fact that the parade of experts he had on his show all believed that the way most Americans were eating and how they lived were at the root of all disease and poor health. Gary Null and his colleagues spoke about the link between diet and depression and how stress can impair our immune systems. They also talked about how factors such as urban living, food allergies, unhealthy relationships, and a feeling of dissatisfaction with our life choices can seriously impair our health. I felt like a veil had been lifted, and I began to see the world, and the choices I had made, in a new way.

I used my lunch hours to visit the local branch of the New York Public Library, and I read every book on nutritional theory and alternative health that I could get my hands on. I also read books about environmental politics and cooking and career building. Without even knowing it, my search for a new life had begun.

I'm not sure why I tuned in to Gary Null's program, except that, on some level, it reminded me of my childhood lifestyle and it comforted me. It brought back memories of the seasonal foods my parents grew and cooked with such loving care, and how marvelous I felt when I enjoyed a diet that was built around homegrown berries, herbs, vegetables, and grains.

After one particularly bad week, when I felt severely depressed and lethargic and had had three migraines in a row, I decided I had to do something, so I picked up the phone and called Gary Null's office. The woman who answered couldn't have been nicer, even though I realize now that I probably sounded like a crazy person to her. I just blurted out that I felt terrible and that I was certain Gary Null could help me. She graciously gave me the name of the doctor who truly changed my life. My first visit with Dr. Christopher Calapai was eye-opening, to say the least. I had never encountered the kinds of therapies he offered, and I was a bit nervous to begin treatment there. Nevertheless, I took a deep breath and decided to hear what he thought, as anything would be better than not knowing what was going on with my body.

I was given skin-prick and kinesiology muscle allergy testing and a detailed nutritional assessment. The results were, at the time, shocking to me. I tested positive for allergies to both wheat and corn, two foods that I ate almost daily, and I had a serious overgrowth of the yeast *Candida albicans* in my system. Dr. Calapai recommended a high-dose multivitamin to help rebuild my immune system, acidophilus and fiber supplements to strengthen my digestive tract, and intravenous vitamin therapy and homeopathic remedies to bring my body back into balance. Then I met with the nutritionist on his staff, who lowered the dietary boom: I had to eliminate sugar (as well as wheat and corn) from my diet. This, they were clear, was nonnegotiable. Up until that point in my life, I would have said, "Forget it!" but I was so miserable and so unwell that I agreed to banish sugar from my diet. To say that I left the office feeling overwhelmed would be an understatement. But I also left that doctor's office feeling something I hadn't felt in a long while: hope.

Never one to work my way into anything gently, I took their recommendations to an extreme. I eliminated dairy, animal products, soda, coffee, wheat, sugar, food additives, and caffeine from my diet. In short, I dove headfirst into my own detox. And it was truly cold turkey. I started to research my food allergies and problems with yeast overgrowth online, and I became immersed in a world that understood that food can either make us healthy or make us sick. I sought out easy-to-prepare recipes that honored all the restrictions and limitations I had to put on my diet. I cobbled together a simple dietary plan that got me on my way as I continued to educate myself about how food can be either our best source of nutritional fuel or the worst kind of pollution we can subject ourselves to.

Changing my diet so radically was the hardest thing I've ever done, but within a week I felt like a new woman. I stopped having headaches, and I woke up each morning more energized and much more alert. I was no longer slipping into a coma after lunch, and I had enough concentration to pursue more in-depth research about dietary theories, food sources, the politics of the food industry, and the powerful effects food marketing has on how we view, eat, and buy food in this country.

Not long after my diet detox, I left the legal office where, I realized, I was just biding my time, and I started working at a job I actually enjoyed. Having been a vintage-store junkie my entire life, I took a job working as an assistant at City Opera Thrift Store in May 2000. I helped organize corporate donations from top designers and fought an endless battle with the mountain of trash bags filled with the castoffs of wealthy New York opera lovers. I had fun at that job, and it energized me while I continued taking my vitamins and working on eating a clean diet. I also started researching cooking schools, where I not only would learn how to cook healthier meals for myself but would be trained to cook like that for others as well.

I wasn't making any money at the thrift store, so I took a night job as a cocktail waitress at a bar in SoHo. I'm not much of a night owl, but this job allowed me to make enough money to start classes at the Natural Gourmet Cookery School, which was founded by Annemarie Colbin in 1977. When I completed the 6-month program, I was awarded an internship as a sous-chef at a macrobiotic restaurant in Milan, Italy. This was a dream come true! Except that I would be leaving New York, a city I had grown to love, as well as my new boyfriend, Morgan. Though I had always been adventurous and eager to try new cities, I had never lived in a foreign country, let alone one where I hardly knew the language. I was also going to Italy to do something that I had never done professionally before, which was to cook for other people. For the first time in my life, I was scared.

Cooking in Milan turned out to be one of the best experiences of my life. I worked 6 days a week under Egyptian chef Mohammed Tourkey. He was a wonderful man, generous and friendly. We worked side by side in the tiny kitchen of *Un Mondo Leggero* (which means "light earth"), creating beautiful organic dishes built around the freshest, most delicious seasonal produce. Our clientele were people who really cared about their health and who were looking to maintain or re-create their health through their diets. The owner of the restaurant is an American man named Martin, who is also a macrobiotic counselor and healer. Although I never fully adopted a "macrobian" lifestyle myself, my time at *Un Mondo Leggero,* working alongside Mohammed and Martin, had a profound influence on my understanding of food and health.

In the midst of my apprenticeship, Morgan came to visit me for a 2-week tour of Italy (joy!), and my virtuous dietary habits went out the window as we explored the sights and restaurants of Venice, Milan, Florence, and Rome. I had been eating primarily whole grains, greens, fruits, and beans, but I gave all that up to gorge on gelato, red wine, pasta and cheese, and anything else that caught our fancy. While my tastebuds said yes, the rest of my body screamed *no!* I contracted a terrible bladder infection and started to have migraines 3 days into our vacation. We spent the rest of our journey finding public restrooms and pharmacies where they sold mysterious packets of powder that managed to keep my infection at bay until I got back to Milan.

When my internship ended, I went back to New York and took a job as a pastry chef at an organic restaurant for several months while I looked for a job that would better match my own cooking ambitions. I didn't just want to cook for people whom I'd never know, I realized; I wanted to cook for people who wanted to find their way back to—or discover for the first time—a truly healthy way of eating. I wanted to help people detox themselves from sugar, caffeine, and the other substances we pollute our bodies with. But I didn't just want to feed these people. I wanted to teach them how to feed themselves. I was driven by the transformation I had seen in my own life. As my overall health had improved, so did other areas of my life. Once I detoxed, I found meaningful work, and I found love in a truly meaningful relationship. I began to realize that changing my diet not only had a profound effect on my health, but it also had an immeasurably positive effect on my life. I was offered a job as the vegetarian chef for The Hole in the Wall Gang Camp in Ashford, Connecticut. This amazing year-round camp, founded by Paul Newman in 1988, supports children with life-threatening illnesses and their families. It was a powerful experience preparing organic menus every day for 60 to 80 people, and it confirmed for me that helping other people eat for health was the direction I wanted to move in. But I wasn't quite getting the personal connection I wanted from this experience. I loved everyone around me, but I was cooking for such a crowd that I simply didn't have the time to get to know any of them. I realized that I wanted to work more directly with individuals. I wanted to work intimately with a person, one on one. That's when I decided to become a personal chef.

I came back to New York and began the legwork of establishing my own business as a personal chef. My first clients were often families with specific health issues: diabetes, cancer, food allergies, and my own favorite, candidiasis. I began working for several families, cooking their meals and tailoring the menus to address their unique needs. I felt proud of my work and liked knowing that I was helping people to feel better while they were learning to eat better. In those early days of building my business, I knew that I needed to learn more about the sophisticated effects nutrition has on wellness. I had seen catalogs for a school called the Institute for Integrative Nutrition, and I had heard good things about it. I attended an orientation session there and realized that this training would beautifully complement my culinary education and would empower me to help my clients in more-meaningful ways. The program offered an in-depth study of nutritional theory, alternative healing, and various counseling techniques. It also brought me into a community of passionate people who care as much about cooking, diet, and health as I do. I learned there that every body is unique and has unique nutritional needs to maintain optimum health. In other words, one diet definitely does not fit all. But the truth that there are basics that benefit us all was something I also learned there.

This book is for everyone who wants to improve his or her health and live a more vibrant, energetic life. *The Great American Detox Diet* is about living and eating with passion and awareness in order to do one thing and one thing only: promote and support excellent health!

# CHAPTER 1

# The All-American Guinea Pig: Morgan's Story

I met Morgan Spurlock in December of 2001, while I was working as a cocktail waitress at night and attending culinary school during the day. He came into the bar one night and we hit it off. The next week, he came in to take me out to breakfast when my shift ended at 4:00 A.M. We have been together ever since, and I have to say that, except for 1 terrifying month, I never gave a thought to the idea that I might lose him. Let me explain.

In 2002, Morgan and I spent Thanksgiving with his family in West Virginia. After another terrific meal (Morgan's mom modified some of her traditional dishes so I could eat them, too), we were watching television and a bizarre news item came on. It seemed that two teenage girls in New York City, who were both quite obese, were suing McDonald's for making them fat and unhealthy. A spokesman for the fast-food industry was speaking out against the lawsuit, and I can still hear him ranting: "You can't link our food to these girls being sick and obese! Our food is healthy, nutritious, and good for you!" I recall being outraged by his comments, and I immediately yelled something back at him, but Morgan's reaction was different. "Wait a minute," he said, "that means I should be able to eat their food for breakfast, lunch, and dinner without any adverse health effects at all." A sense of doom came over me as I turned to him on the couch. But it was too late: The lightbulb had gone off.

Morgan took this contention—that fast food is nutritious and good for you—and put it to the ultimate test. He decided that he would eat only McDonald's food for breakfast, lunch, and dinner for 30 days and record how he felt throughout this monthlong fast-food-only diet. Being a filmmaker, he decided he would make a documentary film about his experience (and, by extension, mine, as a cameraman literally moved into our tiny sixth-floor walk-up apartment for the duration of the project). I remember him laughing at the fact that if nothing bad happened to him, he would be making the greatest advertisement of all time for McDonald's. Unfortunately, this is not what happened at all.

When Morgan began filming *Super Size Me* in early 2003, we had been living together for almost 2 years and he had been eating a diet rich in fresh vegetables, whole grains, fresh fruit, and organic meats and dairy products. Breakfast usually consisted of a fresh fruit shake or a whole grain porridge that was cooked fresh each day, with fruit, nuts, and real maple syrup. (This is a far cry nutritionally from the packets of sweetened oatmeal that you can microwave in 30 seconds: The nutrition in those products has been overshadowed by the unbelievably high amount of sugar that has been added.) For dinner, we always sat down to a home-cooked meal, and I often made a hearty chili or stew, sautéed vegetables with some combination of a whole grain, or beans. Since we both love Mexican food, we occasionally order in from the great restaurant down the block from our apartment. Morgan often ate lunch at his desk or, when he had a meeting, in a restaurant, so he did eat plenty of rich foods such as pasta dishes, meats, and desserts. And he is a card-carrying meat-lover. Even so, his diet (due to the fact that he lived with a vegan chef who loved to cook for him) was nearly two-thirds organic and vegetarian.

For a 33-year-old man, Morgan was in excellent health. He enlisted three well-regarded medical doctors, a nutritionist, and a fitness expert to be a part of his "team" for the month. Fit and trim, he is 6 feet 2 inches and weighed in at 185 pounds, and had only 11 percent body fat. His blood was tested and his cholesterol levels were excellent, as were his other blood levels, including his blood pressure.

He was also physically fit. Morgan (as I had) grew up in an athletic family (he and his two brothers had been—I kid you not—ballet dancers!). He rode his bike all over Manhattan and practiced yoga on a pretty regular basis. He also, like most New Yorkers, walked everywhere. (The average New Yorker walks about 5 miles a day, while citizens in other parts of the country log only 400 yards to 1 mile per day on foot.) The fitness pro told Morgan that both his fitness and flexibility were excellent and that he was in the top 10 percent for his age group in both categories.

I know that I should have been reassured by the fact that Morgan was going into this experiment in superb health, but I couldn't keep my sense of foreboding at bay. Part of what was frightening me was that I was the only one who thought this kind of diet (which, in a relative way, would take the lousy diets most of us have to a surreal extreme) might be seriously bad for Morgan. Not one of the three doctors he consulted suggested that he might jeopardize his health by doing this. They thought he might gain a few pounds and that his cholesterol might rise some, but they all believed that his body would handle it. No problem. How wrong they were, and, sadly, how right I was.

I knew that eating this way would compromise Morgan's health because I had, to a far lesser degree, polluted my own body with fast foods and overprocessed foods before I detoxed myself. I had chosen to make a career out of helping people get away from overly processed foods and feeling bad, and back to a saner, healthier way of eating—which meant going back to fresh, whole foods in their original, un-tampered-with state. There was no way, to my mind, that Morgan would get through this without having to pay a serious price.

Before he got started, Morgan established some simple ground rules. During the 30 days, he vowed to try everything on the menu at least once. And though he would never ask for a meal to be "supersized," if the server offered this option, he had to take it. (During the month, he had nine supersized meals.) He would also monitor how much he walked and would try to walk less, in an effort to mimic the habits of most other Americans. Other than that, all bets were off.

Morgan started his McDonald's odyssey with the glee of a kid who has been let loose in a candy store. He positively bounded into a McDonald's in New York (which has the highest density of McDonald's restaurants per acreage of any city in the United States) and began his new diet. By day 2, after his first supersized meal, he was puking his guts out. At the end of week 1, he had gained an astonishing 9 pounds. Normally energetic, active, and outgoing, he was now cranky and felt lousy enough that he'd arrive home at the end of the day and want to go right to bed.

By the 2nd week, Morgan had gained another 8 pounds, for a total of 17 pounds, which meant that he had gained nearly 10 percent of his body weight! His mood had taken a serious turn for the worse, and he was quite depressed and exhausted by day's end. Also, at this point, his sex drive vanished: It is nearly impossible to feel sexually aroused when you are plagued by headaches, depression, and a feeling of bloated malaise. Despite feeling so bad, Morgan forged ahead and crisscrossed the country, interviewing experts, food industry bigwigs, and people on the street, all the while fueling his body on nothing but McDonald's.

Going into week 3, Morgan's system began to show signs of serious trouble. His percentage of body fat was now 18 percent, and his blood pressure was up, as was his cholesterol. He was struggling to concentrate, often had blinding headaches, and felt depressed and sluggish all the time. (Interestingly, the only thing that would give him a "boost" was eating again, when he'd get a rush from all the caffeine and sugars in the food.) Day 21 was the worst of all: He woke up in the middle of the night with severe pressure in his chest and was having trouble breathing. His doctors recommended that he stop the diet immediately and even advised him, if the pain in his chest persisted, to check into the hospital. At this stage, his blood tests revealed another terrifying development: His liver was beginning to fail, as it had become overwhelmed by the rancid fats he was ingesting. It was toxic and leaking enzymes. The fact that his liver was being destroyed prompted all three of Morgan's doctors to tell him to quit the experiment immediately. (One of his doctors described his liver as being like pâté.) All three of them agreed that what they were seeing mimicked—exactly—what they see in alcoholics who are in the midst of a serious binge. They were now concerned that he would not survive the 30-day McDonald's diet. When Morgan insisted he wouldn't quit, they begged him to at least take an aspirin a day to ward off any heart complications. He declined, saying that taking an aspirin might cloud the results of this experiment, and besides, aspirin wasn't on the menu!

At this point, I felt desperate for him, so I began to plan how I would detox him once he was off this hideous diet.

At the end of week 3, Morgan actually weighed in at a pound lighter, bringing his total weight gain to 16 pounds. His nutritionist reasoned that he had likely lost some muscle mass, given that he was no longer exercising regularly. He was now so fatigued that even climbing the six flights of stairs to our apartment was overwhelming for him, and he'd arrive home pale and out of breath. Nonetheless, he forged on.

Finally, finally day 30 arrived. At his last weigh-in, we learned that he had gained a whopping 24.5 pounds. In one month! His body fat was close to 20 percent, and his cholesterol had gone up 65 points (from 165 to 230). But the numbers were just the half of it. Morgan looked terrible and felt worse. By now, "normal" to him meant feeling depressed, wiped out, and foggy-headed. It was difficult for him to recall feeling fit and well, even though it had been only a month.

Why did McDonald's food make Morgan so sick? Because it is food that is so overly processed and so stuffed with chemicals, fillers, and flavor-enhancers that it has, quite literally, become toxic to us. And I'm not the only one who thinks this.

A study conducted by two prominent physicians in the United States and published in January 2005 in the prestigious British medical journal *The Lancet* shows a correlation between eating fast food and obesity and insulin resistance (a precursor of diabetes). The 15-year study followed 3,000 young Americans and was designed to monitor their cardiac health. Even after making statistical allowances for other factors, the researchers concluded that those who eat fast food two or more times a week are, on average, 10 pounds heavier than those who do not.

"Fast food is commonly recognized to have very poor nutritional quality," stated Dr. David Ludwig, the director of the obesity program at Children's Hospital Boston and the senior author of the study. He continued, "In the absence of such data, the fast-food industry continues to claim that fast food can be part of a healthful diet."

Let's look more specifically at what Dr. Ludwig means by "poor nutritional quality." A man of Morgan's age should take in approximately 2,500 calories a day. No more than 30 percent of his daily intake should be fat, meaning he should not consume more than 68 grams of fat per day. He needs only small amounts of salt in his diet, so sodium intake should be moderate. And he should have stimulants like caffeine and sugar in very low doses, if at all.

Here's what Morgan would ingest—just for breakfast: A Sausage, Egg, and Cheese McGriddle has 560 calories, 32 grams of fat, 1,290 milligrams of sodium, and 16 grams of sugar. Add to this a hash brown, a large coffee with cream, and a large orange juice, and Morgan would consume a breakfast of 895 calories that packed a whopping 41.5 grams of fat (13.5 of which were saturated fats and another 3.5 of which were trans fat, the ticking time bombs that are found only in processed foods), 1,580 milligrams of sodium, and 53 grams of sugar. With breakfast alone, he had met more than a third of his daily caloric needs and more than half of his daily allotment of fat! On top of this, he'd already ingested obscene amounts of salt, sugar, and caffeine. Nutritionally, it was all downhill from here.

On pages 20–21 is a table showing what a typical day for Morgan during his McDonald's-Only Diet might have looked like. Remember that these are foods that McDonald's presents in its advertising as fresh, healthy, and absolutely okay to eat *regularly*. Also, I put this day together based on the McDonald's menu, and it may or may not have been exactly what Morgan ate on any given day, though it does represent, accurately, the nutritional content of his average day.

Since Morgan is about 6 feet 2 inches, keeping his tall frame at a steady weight of 185 would require about 67.8 grams of total fat a day. Based on the sample day on pages 20–21, Morgan could be eating more than twice the amount of fat someone of his height needed for maintaining his weight. According to the National Academy of Sciences, 1,100 to 3,000 milligrams of sodium per day is a healthy range. The McDonald's diet was burying Morgan under twice the recommended amount of sodium to maintain health. The USDA recommends capping added sugar at 6 to 10 percent of daily calories. This diet provided 246 grams of sugar, or 61.5 teaspoons of added sugar a day, which is about 25 percent of the total daily calories.

This all may seem pretty extreme, but remember these are meals that McDonald's presents in its advertising as being *good* for you.

Why is the nutritional content of these "foods" so compromised? Some would argue that it is because they are not foods at all! Instead, they are "food products" that have been modified, formulated, preserved, and marketed to us in such a way that we've been brainwashed into thinking this stuff actually is food and actually is good for us.

Eric Schlosser, in his excellent exposé of the fast-food industry, *Fast Food Nation,* describes in graphic detail how food is formulated and manufactured and shares such tidbits with us as the fact that the aroma from French fries is not a naturally occurring smell—it is basically a perfume that was created in a flavor factory in New Jersey. In essence, these foods—like most foods that come in a box, a bag, or on a frozen tray—have been engineered to appeal to us. These food products have been loaded with ingredients (fat, sugar, salt) and engineered to smell so good that we can't resist them. And that's just what they do.

But fast-food sellers aren't the only ones who are guilty of polluting food with salt and sugar. Just take a look at the "healthful" snacks that await your child on the supermarket shelves. A low-fat, fruit-on-the-bottom yogurt cup has 9½ teaspoons of sugar in it (which is roughly equivalent to the sugar you'd find in 3½ mini candy bars). Pop Tarts, which are sold as a breakfast food, have 32.7 grams of sugar per 100 grams, while Cocoa Puffs have 36.5 grams of sugar per 100-gram serving. This is stuff that is sold as "part of a healthy breakfast" to children all over the United States.

Even I had trouble figuring out what, exactly, was in the food Morgan was eating. Why on earth, I wondered, did something as simple as a fast-food English muffin have more than 30 ingredients in it? And why was there ammonium sulfate in a Big Mac bun? Isn't ammonia a corrosive that is known to burn the eyes, skin, and respiratory tract and that, when ingested in large quantities, can be fatal? What is carboxymethylcellulose gum, and what is it doing in barbeque sauce? Why is sodium aluminum phosphate, a heavy

# A Day in the Life
# of "Super-Size-Me" Morgan

## BREAKFAST

**Sausage, Egg, and Cheese McGriddle:** 560 calories, 32 grams of fat including 1.5 grams of trans fat, 1,290 milligrams of sodium, 16 grams of sugar

**Hash Browns:** 140 calories, 8 grams of fat including 2 grams of trans fat, 290 milligrams of sodium

**Large Coffee with Cream:** 15 calories, 1.5 grams of fat

**Large Orange Juice:** 180 calories, 5 milligrams of sodium, 37 grams of sugar

**Breakfast Total:** 895 calories, 41.5 grams of fat including 3.5 grams of trans fat, 1,585 milligrams of sodium, 53 grams of sugar

## LUNCH

**Quarter Pounder with Cheese:** 510 calories, 25 grams of fat including 1.5 grams of trans fat, 1,150 milligrams of sodium, and 9 grams of sugar

**Large Fries:** 520 calories, 25 grams of fat including 6 grams of trans fat, 330 milligrams of sodium

**Ketchup Packet:** 10 calories, 270 milligrams of sodium, 2 grams of sugar

metal derivative, used as a baking ingredient in chicken nuggets, when aluminum is known to affect nutrient absorption and disrupt organ and nervous system functioning?

No wonder Morgan had so much trouble getting access to nutritional information in the McDonald's stores he visited! There are so many ingredients in these "foods" that they have become unrecognizable to us—and our bodies. But reading the content labels on these products is crucial to our understanding of how toxic these foods truly are.

I realized that Morgan was going to need some serious care and

**Large Coke:** 310 calories, 20 milligrams of sodium, 86 grams of sugar

**Lunch Total:** 1,350 calories, 50 grams of fat including 7.5 grams of trans fat, 1,770 milligrams of sodium, 97 grams of sugar

## DINNER

**Big Mac:** 560 calories, 30 grams of fat including 1.5 grams of trans fat, 1,010 milligrams of sodium, 8 grams of sugar

**Large Fries:** 520 calories, 25 grams of fat including 6 grams of trans fat, 330 milligrams of sodium

**Ketchup Packet:** 10 calories, 270 milligrams of sodium, 2 grams of sugar

**Large Coke:** 310 calories, 20 milligrams of sodium, 86 grams of sugar

**Large Coffee with Cream:** 15 calories, 1.5 grams of fat

**Dinner Total:** 1,415 calories, 56.5 grams of fat including 7.5 grams of trans fat, 1,630 milligrams of sodium, 96 grams of sugar

**Daily Total:** 3,660 calories, 148 grams of fat including 18.5 grams of trans fat, 4,985 milligrams of sodium, 246 grams of sugar

attention to regain his energy, replenish his body, and detoxify his organs and blood. I began to create a diet plan that would remove all the worst parts of the fast-food/processed-food diet and replace them with whole, nutrient-dense foods. Just as fast food had destroyed Morgan's health, I was sure that different foods could—and would—restore his wellness.

Morgan was eating a ridiculously exaggerated version of what is known as (without any irony intended, given its acronym) the Standard American Diet (SAD), which is low in nutrients and high in health-destroyers like sugar, salt, caffeine, and additives. I knew, from my own detox experience, that I would have to work out a plan for Morgan that would undo as much of the damage he'd suffered as possible. To do this, his detox would require a diet that was nearly the opposite of the McDonald's diet. To counter the damage, Morgan would have to eat a plan that had no refined sugar or artificial sweeteners, no animal products or refined carbohydrates, and no caffeine. Why was I going to be so, well, brutal with him? During his 30-day experiment, Morgan ate more than *30 pounds* of sugar, meaning that he ate about 1 pound of various sweeteners a day, including high fructose corn syrup, white cane sugar, and dextrose. The amount of caffeine in McDonald's products isn't published, but according to national standards, each large cup of McDonald's coffee contains 230 to 350 milligrams of caffeine, while every large Coke contains 121 milligrams. By the end of every day, Morgan was getting a huge amount of sugar and caffeine, and the side effects he suffered (headaches, foggy thinking, increased heart rate) can definitely be described as side effects of these stimulants.

I wrote out an 8-week detox diet that I believed would cleanse his body of the harmful fats, toxic residues, and chemicals he had ingested. Plus, it would catapult him into safely and sanely losing the 24.5 pounds he had gained. I packed his diet plan with nutrient-dense and cleansing foods, took away the "trigger foods" like sugar, caffeine, dairy, meat, and wheat, and highlighted several foods that I knew would help his cells to rebuild themselves and repair the damage they had sustained.

The original plan looked like this:

## Morgan's Detox Diet

### NO!

- Sugar
- Refined carbohydrates (white bread, white sugar, white rice)
- Coffee
- Caffeine
- Alcohol
- Dairy
- Meat

## YES!

- 10 to 14 glasses of filtered water a day
- Whole grains: brown rice, millet, quinoa, oats
- Nuts and seeds
- Phytochemical-rich foods: blackberries, blueberries, raspberries, strawberries, watermelon, peaches, plums, sea veggies, cabbage, tomatoes, soy products
- Beans and legumes
- Acidophilus to replenish good bacteria in intestines
- Focus on organic, fresh foods
- Liver-supportive herbs and greens: chicory, escarole, dandelion greens, watercress, endive, arugula, radicchio, broccoli rabe, dandelion root, licorice root, gingerroot

Morgan did experience some serious withdrawal symptoms for the first 3 days, but he also began to feel better. His skin improved, his energy evened out, and after 8 weeks his liver function, blood pressure, cholesterol levels, and mental attitude all came back to normal. At first, we wanted to see how well he would do on the detox without restoring his healthy lifestyle habits (such as biking and exercising), and we were pleased to see that, after 8 weeks of only changing his diet, he lost 10 pounds. He also began to feel like his old, energetic self again. His headaches didn't return, and his depression lifted. We even found our bedroom rhythm again.

For the next weeks and months, as Morgan resumed his "normal" life and began to exercise again, he continued to lose weight at a steady, slow, and healthy pace. He also made the transition through his detox and found his way back into a healthy, wholesome, and natural way of eating that he continues to this day. It no longer entails me making lists of good foods and forbidden foods: It has become a way of life for him. And when you detox, you will change your life, too.

Since *Super Size Me* premiered in May 2004, I have received more than 70,000 hits on my Web site and hundreds of e-mails from all over the United States from people wanting to "detox the way Morgan did." I read so many stories of bad health, depression, and desperation from so many of you who want to cleanse your bodies and restore yourselves to a healthy way of eating. It is you who have inspired me to write this book.

# CHAPTER 2

# The Sad, Sad American Diet

The criticism of *Super Size Me* was sharp: "No one eats fast food every meal of every day—no wonder Morgan gained all that weight!" Fast-food executives and lobbyists ran to the media shouting foulplay and pointed to an unfair examination of their industry. "Our customers make healthy choices—just look at our new salads menu!" was another battle cry. Yes, McDonald's sold more than 150 million salads in 2003. This seems like a huge number—and might lead one to believe that Americans are finally making healthy choices at fast-food outlets. But you have to look only a bit closer at the numbers to realize that, though we're moving in the right direction when we order a salad, not really very many of us have budged yet. Every day, McDonald's serves more than 46 million people—that means the 150 million salads sold in 2003 represent less than 1 percent of the total annual sales.

But we're not just eating poorly when we go to McDonald's or any other fast-food restaurant. We Americans, who live in the richest country on Earth, have a terribly poor diet. Why is that? What is it about the Standard American Diet (SAD) that is so toxic? The SAD is high in animal and unhealthy hydrogenated fats, and low in fiber and complex carbohydrates. The SAD includes mostly highly processed foods and is low in plant-based foods—all the dietary factors that are known to increase the risk of the most-common modern American diseases, such as cancer, heart disease, and stroke. Our most consumed "vegetable" is the French fry, and according to the Food and Drug Administration, the average American ate about two-thirds of a cup of sugar a day in 2001, which is much higher than the daily limit recommended by the USDA of 10 teaspoons of added sugar.

Okay. So most of us do not eat three meals a day from a drive-thru. But many of us do open a frozen carton, a vacuum-sealed bag, or a cardboard box each day and don't do much more in the kitchen than boil some water or press "start" on the microwave. It's almost impossible not to eat fast food these days—airports are filled with food-chain outlets, and highway off-ramps are full of fast-food places, not organic, whole food markets. We're bombarded with media messages every day telling us that eating something fun and easy will chase our blues away and get us off our feet and onto the couch as quickly as possible. (Sometimes I think that throwing away the television would be the best way to drown out the voices encouraging us to just give in and enjoy a break today!)

Why, then, are we killing ourselves with the Standard American Diet, even when our own government is now telling us not to?

Nearly half a century ago, the United States government drew up a guide to healthy eating that eventually evolved into the food pyramid the USDA promotes today. The goal of the pyramid is to visually help us understand what types of food we should eat in abundance and what types of food we should avoid. Even with this ubiquitous graphic, we ignored the government's advice and continued to eat too much of the wrong things. In early 2005, outgoing Health and Human Services Secretary Tommy Thompson radically revised the government's daily food intake suggestions (they may no longer look like a pyramid) and stunned the nation—including people in the health care industry—when he bluntly stated that Americans have to eat fewer calories and exercise more (he advocated for 60 to 90 minutes a day) if we are going to stop the obesity epidemic. Citing the fact that two out of three Americans are overweight, Thompson said, "It's really common sense. Do you want to look better? Do you want to feel better? You lower your calorie intake, you lower your carbs, your fats. You eat more fruits and vegetables, and you exercise." He urged people to focus on whole foods, particularly whole grains, vegetables, and fruits. He also urged citizens to cut their carbohydrate intake and to limit intake of bad fats, cholesterol, sugar, salt, and alcohol. What was striking about his announcement is that he admitted, though in a rather circumspect way, that all of us will have to work hard to eat around the aggressive marketing of the food industry, which saturates us (especially kids) with advertising for unhealthy food products. "We in this administration feel strongly that people should have an opportunity to advertise," Thompson said. "But we have to do a better job to get out and more aggressively tell the other side." He also did us all a favor by resisting using the word "serving," which has utterly lost its meaning in this age of ridiculous supersizing. Instead, he talked about food intake in terms of cups and ounces, and calories.

The USDA originally created the first food pyramid in the 1960s, due to the skyrocketing rates of heart disease in this country. Even back then, our own government saw that the Standard American Diet was a major factor in causing serious diseases. By 1994, the Nutrition Labeling and Education Act was enacted, and every food product sold from the shelves of our supermarkets was, by law, required to come with important nutritional information on the packaging. These were steps in the right direction, but many of us are still confounded and struck dumb by the barrage of advertising we're fed that contradicts what is on food labels. We're also buried by thousands of fad diets each year and by the conflicting information we get from the government, the food industry, and various special interest groups. Our heads are so busy spinning that we've forgotten to eat right and exercise regularly.

There was a time, of course, before the Industrial Revolution and the birth of the modern food industry, that was built on the concept of mass production, when we did eat whole foods that are nutrient dense. But over the last century, we've moved further and further from eating and preparing whole, fresh foods. In fact, we've become so reliant on the convenience of processed foods that many of us have simply forgotten how to eat right.

And this isn't just an American problem. In most places around the world, people have traditionally eaten the bounty of the local landscape. (I've included an overview of traditional international diets in the resource section of this book.) But in a world that prides itself on rapid globalization, we're all beginning to eat the same diet. The Standard American Diet is, quite tragically, rapidly becoming the Standard World Diet. And it is time for a global wake-up call.

Most cultures around the world used to build their diets around seasonal, fresh whole foods. I say "used to," because there is now hardly a corner of the globe that hasn't been invaded by the modern Western diet and its attendant "illnesses of excess" that plague us today: diabetes, heart disease, cancer, obesity.

In the 1920s and '30s, Dr. Weston Price, a dentist, spent years traveling around the globe, visiting and studying indigenous cultures. His findings were stunning. In many multigenerational families, Dr. Price saw the overall health of offspring deteriorate when a Western-style diet of refined flour and sugar was introduced. Facial and jaw structures narrowed, diseases appeared as if out of thin air, and mental retardation began to affect the younger generations. Their new diets were changing centuries of healthy bone structure and creating disease. The incidences of kidney stones, diabetes, obesity, cancer, and heart disease are on the rise in Japan since the 1950s, when that country was first exposed to a Western-style diet. Their once vegetable-rich diet is now centered more around animal protein, refined carbohydrates, sugar, and fat, just like America's.

Food can hurt us or heal us, and given what's happening to us on the current SAD, it is, frankly, now killing us. The SAD is full of foods that are toxic to our bodies and minds because it is a diet comprised of mostly refined, overly processed, and mass-manufactured food. It is the very concept of convenience (think microwave, drive-thru, or anything that you can carry in your bag without it melting, spoiling, or rotting, and you'll start to get the picture) that has gotten us into such nutritional trouble. A recent reality show from the BBC in England vividly illustrated how hard it is to get around eating "prepared" foods. A family of four was banned from shopping at their supermarket for 2 weeks—how would they do without their favorite foods? For the first time in years, the family was forced to cook from scratch—no boxed, canned, frozen, or prepared foods were allowed. It was a difficult transition for them, especially the mother, who shouldered most of the cooking responsibility. She soon learned that special trips to the local butcher, the kitchen supply store, and the green grocer were necessary. This family didn't own most of the basic kitchen tools one needs for preparing a meal, and even making a pot of tea from loose tea leaves was a challenge for them. But this family, sadly, is not exceptional. They represent most of us. It has become almost impossible to see (isn't that the point of convenience?), but we've become absolutely reliant on time-saving, prepackaged foods, while we've all but forgotten the one skill that is truly basic to human survival—how to prepare and cook our own food.

One of the great ironies of this situation lies in our status as the wealthiest nation on Earth. Here we are, with the financial resources to farm organically, to invest in the research and development to come up with alternatives to using chemicals, sugars, and other additives to make processed foods palatable (if the auto industry can move toward a more environmentally friendly model with hybrid cars, why can't the food industry do the same?), to feed ourselves well instead of stuffing ourselves to death. Instead, we're spending that wealth on medical care to combat the diseases (obesity, diabetes, heart disease) that are the direct result of the SAD.

The fast-food lifestyle is cheap—on the surface. But the costs over the long term of eating a diet like this are incalculable. Prices stay low because the minimum-wage workers McDonald's employs are discouraged from unionizing for better pay, and farmers are given bottom dollar for their mass-produced meat and grains by the huge global food companies that profit enormously from the sheer volume of "food products" we consume. Our reliance on the SAD deprives us of fresh, vital foods and has also severed our connection to a vital and important community. Small family farmers are almost extinct, and the cheap commodity foods that we buy encourage, support, and maintain this system that has a stranglehold on our food chain from seed to field to table.

Most of us just don't know how incompatible most of the foods in the SAD are with the human body—they're so overprocessed, so full of preservatives and chemicals, that they've become void of the natural energy that fresh, whole foods provide. Most egregiously, they seriously corrupt the digestive system, which is the only way the body has to process foods and find nutrition.

The food chain in America continues to grow longer and with more processing, shipping, and other steps involved in getting food from the field to the plate. With every addition to this chain, there is another opportunity for something to go wrong with our food. Highly processed food is difficult to digest. It overtaxes our systems in ways that most of us are unaware of. Modern convenience foods are engineered to ensure consistent taste, texture, and uniformity of shape. They are designed to withstand the bruising of shipping and handling, and to enjoy a long shelf life. The food industry loads them with chemical additives that make the original food all but unrecognizable. There are additives for stability, soy proteins for restoring texture, emulsifying gums to stop separation of ingredients, and sweeteners and flavors to make up for a lack of, well, *flavor*.

Though the number of links in the food chain seems only to grow, the number of companies that supply this food is shrinking, as huge food conglomerates have a stranglehold on our consumption. Americans buy 50 percent of their food products from only 10 companies. It is the government's job to keep an eye on these giant food manufacturers and to make sure that the food sold in supermarkets is safe. Yet it is the FDA who has admitted that about one billion pounds of chemical additives are put into our foods every year and that the average American eats more than 50 pounds of additives a year.

The FDA says it "evaluates all food additives for safety before they are allowed in foods and has found them to be safe and effective in the quantities in which they are consumed in foods." This testing is performed to give additives an approval label of *GRAS*, which means "generally recognized as safe." While the small amounts of single additives found in processed foods are tested as safe, there have been no long-term studies to determine what effect these chemicals have on our bodies over a span of years. Food additives are not tested for their ability to build up in our systems over time, nor are they tested in terms of how they react with other *GRAS* chemicals that are in the foods we eat.

McDonald's and other fast-food companies have used these additives to create attractive, good-smelling foods that can be produced quickly and cheaply all over the world. Little did we know that Morgan would be consuming things like diacetyl tartaric acid esters of fatty acids, polysorbate 20, and sodium stearoyl lactylate. He also ate propylene glycol alginate, monosodium glutamate (or MSG), nitrates, nitrites, and a whole rainbow of food colorings. The effects these chemicals had on his body were obvious.

Not only was he overdosing on calories, but he was also overdosing on substances that were making it difficult for his body to maintain itself on the cellular level.

Morgan was eating only highly processed food, and it was destroying him metabolically. What does this mean? When we refer to someone's metabolism, we're not just talking about whether or not that person is skinny or fat. *Metabolism,* which comes from the Greek word for change, is the uptake and digestion of nutrients and food and the disposal of waste from our bodies. When our metabolic processes are working well, our food gets digested, nutrients get properly distributed to our cells, and our bodies run like well-oiled machines.

Cells are the most basic structures of human life. They are versatile and do everything for us: They gather energy from nutrients and are the building blocks for all of our organs, our blood, our skeletons, and our skin. Cells repair damage, fight germs, and transmit crucial information from one part of the body to another. Our cells extract the nourishment they need for functioning once the food we've ingested has gone through the process of digestion.

What is digestion, and how does the body digest food, anyway? Digestion is the process by which the body breaks down food into individual nutrients that can be used by the body's myriad cells. It all begins in the mouth with teeth and saliva. Chewing is the most important step of digestion, though most of us barely chew our food at all. Chewing is crucial to healthy digestion because it prompts the release of enzymes in our saliva that actually prep the food for further breakdown once it enters our bodies. So if we're not chewing our food and mixing it with adequate saliva, the entire digestive process is compromised. When this happens, we limit the body's ability to extract the nutritional and energy components of food effectively. And isn't that why we're eating in the first place, to fuel our bodies? The enzymes contained in our saliva moisten the food for easier movement, and they begin the digestion of fats and starches. So Mom was right—chew your food! And, I'd add, chew it well: By chewing each mouthful of food until it is almost liquid, you will ease digestion and get as many nutrients out of your food as possible.

Once we begin chewing our food, the stomach receives messages that food is on the way, and it begins to secrete acids that will help to digest protein and further break down fat. This acidic environment of the stomach is an inhospitable environment for bacteria, so keeping our stomachs happy and healthy (and producing wonderful digestive acids) is one of our best lines of defense against any dangerous microorganisms that might enter the gastrointestinal system through the mouth.

The lower part of the stomach is where a lot of movement and action happens—the food, now mixed up with enzymes and acids, gets ground up and moved into the small intestine. This is where healthy intestines become really important: The middle section of the small intestine, called the jejunum, is where most nutrients are absorbed into the body. Amino acids and most vitamins and minerals are absorbed in the inner folds of the intestines by the little hairy *villi* and *microvilli* that populate the bumpy, curved lining of these tubes. Fiber from plant-based foods is indigestible, so it moves right through this area of the intestines, acting as a scrub brush and moving any old bits of food along through the intestines as waste. Really getting rid of this waste is what keeps the intestines clean and running smoothly. The small intestine also works to absorb dietary fat by using bile (which breaks down fat) that is produced by the liver and stored in the gall bladder.

It probably goes without saying, but what we eat determines how well our digestion works. Eating a diet loaded with fat can overtax the liver and gall bladder, while eating a diet high in sugar can overwhelm even the strongest stomach and give rise to the growth of unhealthy bacteria in the intestines. This is one of the hidden ailments that plagued me before my own detox, in the form of *Candida albicans,* and it is my belief that many of us (given our high-sugar diets and overuse of antibiotics, which kill the good bacteria) are walking around with too much of this yeast in our intestines. Every human intestine on the planet contains good and bad bacteria. The friendly bacteria, called acidophilus, are responsible for keeping the colon healthy by causing fermentation and keeping the unhealthy *Candida albicans* bacteria from taking over. An overgrowth of bad bacteria can lead to a myriad of health problems, such as bloating, diarrhea, indigestion, yeast infections, and headaches. But these ailments can be eliminated when one eats a sugar-free, balanced diet.

To make any detox work, it only makes sense to do the food preparation yourself at home, and for Morgan, this aspect of the detox brought him back down to earth in really important ways. He had forgotten, in just 30 short days, how pleasurable it was to sit at a table and just relax and partake of simple, beautifully and lovingly prepared foods that looked and smelled so delicious to him. And to regain the peace of mind that knowing where those foods come from (the earth, not the laboratory!) brings.

Once Morgan's detox was under way and he was beginning to feel better, he was able to look beyond just the dietary aspects of it and begin to add back detoxifying, health-boosting lifestyle elements, such as exercise, adequate rest, and (most important) the renewing of his relationships with friends and loved ones.

One of the great things that came out of the success of *Super Size Me* was that Morgan was able to draw attention to the terrible epidemic of obesity in the United States in ways that our health care givers just haven't been able to. Morgan is just a regular guy who did us all a favor by asking food industry leaders, doctors, educators, and policy makers tons of tough questions. Then he set it all to music and made it fun to watch. By doing this, he opened our eyes to the truth about the Standard American Diet. He also gave me the opportunity to lead him through a successful detox, and now I have the chance to share the wisdom and benefit of detoxing with all of you.

# CHAPTER 3

# Why Americans Need to Detox— Not Diet

**Someone's got to say it,** and I'm sorry it's got to be me: We are the fattest nation on the planet. According to the Centers for Disease Control and Prevention, more than 60 percent of the American population is overweight. That means that two out of three of us are consuming too much of the wrong kinds of food. And the scary part of this statistic is that the fastest-growing segment of the population that is becoming obese is our kids. This means that diseases that once affected only adults, such as heart disease, diabetes, and cancer, are turning up in people who are younger and younger. This is why the obesity problem in the United States has been called an epidemic.

Paradoxically, Americans also spend more than $33 billion on dieting products and services each year, even while the obesity epidemic grows at alarming rates. It has been estimated that 50 million Americans are on some kind of "diet" at all times, but research shows that the vast number of diets fail over the long term (most dieters manage to lose some or all of the weight they'd hoped to, but they quickly replace the pounds or even add to them once they stop the diet of choice). This is why most dietitians and nutritionists in this country feel like they're waging such a losing battle: Most of their patients and clients are busy yo-yoing on one fad diet or another and so neglect to look at the larger picture of how their eating habits affect their health and wellness.

I hate the word *diet* because it is so misused and misunderstood in this country. The reason we spend so much money on "dieting" in the first place is because the Standard American Diet—which, let's be clear, is a diet—is making us all so sick. This is one of the things about Americans that I just don't understand: We ignore what we are putting into our mouths on a daily basis until we are either fat or feel terrible, or both. Then we decide we will pay attention and begin to "diet." Yet so few of us want to acknowledge the poor diets that we live by day in and day out that brought us to such a sorry state of health in the first place. In my professional life, I've learned that using the word *diet* only brings on anxiety for most of my clients. Instead, we talk about food and eating and nutrition and health. Diet just doesn't cut it anymore. That's why I prefer that we think about detoxing instead.

The concept of detoxing is pretty intense. Most of us equate it with kicking drugs or alcohol, and the word invokes images of people writhing on beds riding out delirium tremens, or DTs (cold sweats, tremors, vomiting, delirium), or locked up in prisonlike detox centers, or spending all their time in 12-step meetings. In short, we think of detoxing as the use of an extreme method for eliminating a toxic substance from our bodies. This is absolutely what detoxing is—in part. But detoxing, once you get past the initial elimination of the harmful substance, is also a gentle method of cleansing and a noninvasive way of rebalancing. It is the departure point for rejuvenation and the restoration of our health, vitality, and wellness. I think of detoxing as a beginning and not as the end.

It has always struck me as odd that Americans will spend money on pills, surgery, or some other kind of invasive procedure to remedy the damage wrought by their diets, rather than follow the noninvasive, holistic approach to healing that is the foundation of detoxing. In my practice, I see that this is slowly beginning to change, and it is my hope that this book will serve to accelerate that change.

Given how we Americans currently eat, and how harmful and polluting so much of what we put into our bodies is, *detox* is absolutely the right word for what I'm promoting. Sure, the detox I propose might bring on some side effects (Morgan really did feel awful at first without all that caffeine and sugar pumping through his system), but often these early side effects are nothing more than an indicator of how truly toxic things have become within.

Part of the reason we all need to detox is that our bodies (especially our livers and kidneys) have become saturated with toxins that we've absorbed over time through the air we breathe, the fluids we drink, and the food we eat. Toxins can be poisons, heavy metals, pesticides, fungicides, cleaning solvents, smog, and many substances that we don't even know are leeching into our bodies via our clothing, our furniture, and even our carpets. Many of the worst toxins we can ingest are put into our foods as additives and preservatives, yet most of us aren't even aware of this.

When your body encounters toxins, it has only a few ways to handle them: It hides them in fat; dumps them into tissue, such as muscle, organs, and bone; or eliminates them through waste. An overloaded body will alert you that it is in a toxic state by sending out messages in the form of fatigue, gas, headaches, food cravings, constipation, food allergies, chronic pain, blood sugar imbalances such as diabetes and hypoglycemia, attention problems, premenstrual syndrome, poor sleep, acne and other skin problems, poor digestion, bad breath, and a host of other conditions.

Watching Morgan's body and spirit deteriorate so quickly during his 30-day fast-food diet prompted me into action—what could I do to help him regain his energy and health? I was reminded of how my own ill health had propelled me to radically change my diet 4 years before, and I began to realize that a similar kind of detox would work for Morgan. I sat down at the computer and started typing away, while Morgan sat at the other end of the room, drowning his sorrows in yet another large soda.

There were six main areas of his fast-food diet that were hurting Morgan: He wasn't hydrated enough; he was eating too much sugar and refined carbohydrate; he was getting too much caffeine; he was getting too much fat; he was getting too much protein; and he wasn't getting enough fiber or vitamins and minerals to sustain proper body function. It was incredible that Morgan could be eating so many calories a day—nearly twice the recommended amount—but could still be craving snacks and feeling hungry all the time. I saw that his body wasn't crying out for more fat, sugar, caffeine, and protein—his body was getting plenty of those. What his body really wanted and needed were minerals, vitamins, and vibrant, fresh foods. His body was calling out for healthful meals, not another un-happy meal.

The detox diet I was creating began to take shape. The focus was to reduce and eventually eliminate the foods and ingredients that were harming Morgan's body, while also giving him the foods and nutrients that his body so desperately needed for healing. I had learned, from my own experience, that a true detox involves not just removing the harmful aspects of a diet and lifestyle but replacing those toxins with healthy foods and new, more beneficial ways of approaching life.

Nutrient-dense seasonal produce as well as simple, whole foods would be the foundation of Morgan's recovery. And once his body was on the mend, we'd work on rebalancing his lifestyle, too.

I had also learned that an effective detox is not just about eating food. Connecting with your food by shopping for it and cooking it will help give you more control over your detox, and these activities will help you listen better to your body and what it needs.

To help you determine if you would benefit from a detox diet, I've put together a series of questions that are designed to get you thinking much more consciously about your diet and lifestyle. See "A Questionnaire: Do I Need to Detox?" on pages 38 to 39.

While he was on the McDonald's diet, poor Morgan would have answered yes to all the questions that point to him not feeling well. Many of my clients who suffer from serious chronic diseases such as diabetes come to me feeling just as terrible as Morgan did. All of them, regardless of how severe their unwellness is at the outset, report feeling remarkably clearer, less "stopped up," and more energetic once they've gone through the detox.

## WHY THE DETOX DIET IS PRESENTED IN 8-WEEK INCREMENTS

The reason the detox diet is broken down into 8-week chunks is actually quite simple. It took exactly 8 weeks for Morgan to regain his normal body functions and blood levels after the McD's diet. I've also learned, through my own detox and working with my clients, that it takes at least a week to feel the effects of giving up a toxic food or substance and to get to the other side of any withdrawal symptoms one might have. In other words, if you are going to quit sugar or caffeine or make a significant and lasting dietary change, you'll need a week to let your brain say goodbye to the bad and hello to the new.

## A QUICK OVERVIEW OF MORGAN'S DETOX

The main points of Morgan's detox diet correspond to what is most out of balance with the typical Standard American Diet. Flushing his body with more-natural liquids, especially water, was the first step to detoxifying his system. In addition, many of us are self-medicating with high doses of caffeine and sugar to get us through our stressful days and to help us cope with our unfulfilling life choices. Though Morgan loves his work and tends to be a pretty easygoing guy, during his 30-day fast-food diet, Morgan's body became overloaded with these stimulants, and they took a terrible toll on his normally even-keeled mood and high energy levels. So getting him off sugar and caffeine (which caused terrible withdrawal symptoms at first) were the next steps in his detox.

Because the digestive and intestinal tracts are really the seat of health, adequate fiber intake is crucial in order to keep things moving. According to the National Health and Nutrition Examination Survey, people in the United States get just 30 percent of the fiber they need each day. I can't stress enough how truly bad this is for everyone's health—and for a successful detox. Focusing on whole grains and the healthy complex carbohydrates found in vegetables and fruits boosted Morgan's fiber intake and gave his digestive system necessary support so it could begin to eliminate the toxins he had ingested. Morgan had also eaten way too much fat and protein on the McD's diet, and so I steered him away from dairy products and meat; this allowed his body to reduce the stress that the high protein consumption had put on his already overtaxed organs. Dairy is one of the top food allergens, and the meats we consume on the SAD are all too often contaminated

*(continued on page 40)*

## A QUESTIONNAIRE: DO I NEED TO DETOX?

The goal of this questionnaire is to help you think with more precision and clarity about your diet and how you feel. Take a look at your answers and see if they are related to how you feel.

### CURRENT DIET

- Do you use sugar and/or caffeine often as a "pick-me-up"?
- Do you eat a diet high in processed, refined foods?
- What types of carbohydrates do you eat? How often?
- Do you drink sodas and sweetened sports drinks?
- Do you snack mindlessly throughout the day?
- Do you eat more than three servings of protein a day?
- Do you eat fish? How often? What types of fish?
- Do you eat more than 6 eggs a week?
- Do you eat French fries, potato chips, fried fish, or fried eggs? How often?
- Do you eat nuts and seeds? What kinds? How often?
- How many servings of vegetables do you eat a day?
- How many servings of fruit do you eat a day?
- Do you enjoy cooking?
- How often do you cook your own food or eat homemade meals?

### CURRENT PHYSICAL STATE

- Are you overweight or obese?
- Do you get headaches?
- Do you get bloated or have cramps after eating?
- Do you have problems with diarrhea and/or constipation?
- Are your nails and hair strong and pliable?
- Do you use or abuse alcohol or cigarettes?
- Do certain foods make you tired or cranky?
- Do you have asthma, hay fever, rashes, or environmental allergies?
- How are your teeth? Do you have several fillings? What color are they?
- Do you have food allergies?
- Do you have high blood pressure and/or high cholesterol?

- Do you have acne?
- What health problems have your parents had?
- Women: Are your periods painful?
- Do you have mood swings before or during menstruation?
- Have you skipped your menstrual cycle for a period longer than 3 months?

## CURRENT ENERGY LEVEL

- Do you feel awake and refreshed when wake?
- Do you feel stagnant in your life and energy?
- Do you feel "stuck" in your body?
- Do you often feel tired and foggy in the middle of the day?

## CURRENT LEVEL OF PHYSICAL EXERCISE

- Do you exercise as much as you would like to?
- Do you experience shortness of breath when you exercise?
- Do you exercise for at least 30 minutes 5 or more days of the week?
- What are your reasons for not exercising more?
- Is exercise a fun activity for you?
- Do you enjoy playing team sports, or do you prefer single-person activities?
- Were you encouraged to be physically active when you were growing up?
- Did your parents enjoy sports or exercising?
- Does exercise relax you, or does it make you tired?

## CURRENT METABOLIC STATE

- After a meal of mostly protein, do you feel tired or bloated?
- Do you feel better when you eat fewer carbohydrates and more protein?
- Are you slender, plump, or very large?
- Is your skin thin and dry, hot and oily, or thick and cold?
- Are you always hungry, or can you skip meals?
- Are you always thirsty?
- Do you have constipation or diarrhea often?

with hormones and antibiotics, which are known to destroy the healthy intestinal bacteria that is so important to digestion and to maintaining a healthy immune system. Focusing on tasty, non-animal sources of protein allowed Morgan's body to have a chance to heal and rebuild. Finally, adding back in many nutrient-dense fresh fruits, vegetables, herbs, and spices replenished his depleted body. By following my detox program, Morgan was, very quickly, able to undo all the damage he had done to his body. I'm certain that in detoxifying your own diet, you will regain health and vitality, too.

Before we move onto the 8-week program, I want to give you a quick walk through the major nutritional areas that we will cover.

# Detox Overview: What We'll Tackle

## Water

Getting back to basics is a major part of this detox plan. The simple truth is that the human body has not evolved as drastically as the world we have built around ourselves, and our bodies need and thrive on simple foods and nourishment. Our bodies do not *need* caffeine and sugar—these are foods and substances that are relatively new to our culture in the huge amounts that we consume them in. Traditional cultures all over the world remain healthy and free of our chronic, preventable diseases mainly because their diets are simple, fresh, local, and seasonal.

Chapter 4 details why water is so important to human health. Tips for integrating more water into your day will help fill the gap for those of us who "just don't like water." This detoxification process is about removing the negative and adding positive steps—using water as a first step to flush out, clean up, and fill up is really important.

## Sugar

When did saccharin and "maple-flavored syrup" become necessary to human existence? The global supermarket has evolved to supply us with our every wish, any day of the year. Sugar used to be just that—sugar. Until a few decades ago, the only sugars found in homes and bakeries were the white sugar derived from crushing the liquid out of cane stalks, honey, maple syrup, and a few other minor sweeteners like agave nectar. Besides the countless calorie-free artificial sweeteners such as aspartame and saccharin, food manufacturers use high fructose corn syrup, fructose, xylitol, mannitol, isomalt, lactilol, erythritol, sorbitol, and maltitol. Our food is sweet, and our health has gone sour because of it.

Rethinking our love affair with sugar is an important part of detoxifying and healing our bodies from all sorts of medical concerns. Chapter 5 will explain how sugar is hurting our bodies, and how so many of us use it as an emotional crutch to deal with other areas of our lives that are painful or unsatisfying. Sugar's powerful properties are important to understand, and Morgan and I are both examples of how kicking a sugar addiction can practically save your life.

## Caffeine

Caffeine is an addictive substance—no question about that. Talking with friends and clients over the years about caffeine has always brought up the idea that it is something to be "used." Some of us are able to "use" this additive to get through a rough day at work when we didn't sleep well or to help us stay up late to finish a project. Incredible numbers of Americans die every year from diseases associated with caffeine stimulation, such as heart disease, high blood pressure, anxiety, and depression, yet government and industry regulations don't try to shield us from the harm being poured into our morning cup. Cardiovascular disease is the number one killer in the United States. In 2000, nearly one million Americans died of heart disease, which means that 40 percent of all deaths that year were caused by cardiovascular diseases. Studies have shown that several factors contribute to most heart attacks: smoking, abnormal lipoprotein ratios, diabetes, high stress-hormone levels, and high blood pressure. Consuming a lot of caffeine affects cholesterol levels adversely and also contributes to high blood pressure, higher stress-hormone levels, and higher homocysteine, all of which are known to contribute to an increased risk of heart attack.

Morgan's diet was loaded with extra caffeine from the sodas that he drank every day. The average American drinks two 8-ounce servings of soda a day. With each can of soda (12 ounces) containing between 37 and 71 milligrams of caffeine, it's little wonder that so many people's hearts are exhausted. The average consumption for teenaged boys is three cans or more of soda daily. Removing caffeine from your diet will take a lot of stress off of vital organs and body functions. Chapter 6 details further issues concerning caffeine consumption and offers concrete ways to reduce your need and finally eliminate this additive before it does any more harm to your body.

## Fat

This detoxification is not about weight loss—it is about removing the negative toxins that accumulate in our bodies due to our environment, diet, and lifestyle. However, because many toxins are fat-soluble, meaning they dissolve in fat and are therefore stored and found in our fatty tissues, losing weight will automatically reduce the amount of toxins your body is storing. The wonderful thing about this detoxification diet is that it provides the body with a healing amount of nutrition while reducing the amount of calories normally contained in the SAD, leading to automatic weight loss.

A fast-food SAD diet, like the one Morgan ate for a month, is full of fats, which are necessary for life. Fat makes food taste good, it cushions our cells and organs, and it helps us to utilize important nutrients in our bodies. However, an overload of fat in our diets, especially dangerously manufactured fats such as hydrogenated and trans fat, can cause serious health problems. Chapter 7 explains more fully the role of fat in our bodies and diet, as well as tips for using healthier types of cooking oils and avoiding bad fat in foods.

## Whole Grains and Complex Carbohydrates

Carbohydrates give us energy—but they can also bulk up our bodies if they're refined and stripped of their whole, natural qualities.

White flour and bread products were developed for a specific reason in our modern supermarkets: shelf life. Bugs and mice know they can't live on refined white flour products, so these foods tend to stay "good" on the shelf for a long time. Storing whole grain breads and whole flour products is a big concern for a food company because they don't want their products to go bad before someone buys them. By removing the bran and germ of a whole grain, most of the nutrients are stripped away, too—leaving a fluffy white product that must be "enriched" if it is to have any nutritional value at all.

One thing that Morgan's fast-food diet did provide plenty of was carbohydrates—but they were completely refined, and he was getting very little fiber from his food. Nearly all dietary fiber comes from the insoluble structural matter of plants; the fiber a plant uses to keep its stalks and leaves strong and upright provides a structure for its growth, but our digestive systems cannot digest this chewy matter. So when we eat whole grains, fruits, and vegetables, the fiber from these foods passes through our intestines, cleaning us out and keeping things moving. Chapter 8 will focus on the benefits of including complex carbohydrates in your detoxification diet.

## Protein

The fast-food, SAD-style diet that we all know and love is heavily focused on protein. On an average day, Morgan ate a lot of calories, sugar, and fat. But there was one other nutrient that he was overloading his body with, and the serious ramifications of this are widespread throughout the United States. On an average day, Morgan was eating between 65 and 80 grams of protein. Now in this protein-heavy culture we live in, many people would think that this is a good, healthy amount. For some men who are weight lifters, this amount of protein might work just fine. But consider what happened to Morgan's body as he ate this diet.

By the 21st day, Morgan's blood tests showed a huge spike in the level of uric acid in his blood, which was leading his body toward developing hyperuricemia and gout, a painful kind of arthritis. Too much protein, coupled with the inability to digest it, can cause these elevated levels of uric acid in the blood. Interestingly, most fast-food customers are men, and among the male population in the United States, approximately 10 percent have hyperuricemia.

Protein, along with fats and carbohydrates, is a macronutrient vital to human health. But what kind of protein should we be eating? One thing that the USDA food pyramid doesn't address is the question of *quality*—where do your protein sources come from? What hidden ingredients are found in the most-consumed forms of protein? What kind of protein works best for your body? Because you're an individual with specific needs and a unique body, blanket statements about protein intake are not helpful. Chapter 9 is centered around issues of protein needs, possible symptoms of too much or too little protein intake, and ideas for expanding your protein options.

## Beyond Your Diet

As I mentioned earlier in the book, it's not just our food that is toxic to us. We need to look at the larger environment around us and detox as much of that as possible in order to truly reach a state of maximum health and wellness. Chapter 10 focuses on the environmental toxins we need to clear from our lives.

## The Detox Lifestyle

Detoxing is a way of life. Once you've come to understand how great an impact food has on your health and wellness, you can't help but see that what you put into your life beyond food—such as your work, your relationships, your overall activities—also has a great impact on your well-being. Chapter 11 puts it all together and shows you how detoxing your diet is just the first step to living a truly detoxed life.

**PART TWO**

# THE 8-WEEK DETOX PLAN

CHAPTER 4

# Everyone into the Pool!

## Week 1: Getting Your Detox Under Way
## Nutritional Issue: Water

I remember, when I was a child, watching an episode of *Star Trek* in which some alien species was yet again trying to take over the Starship Enterprise. One of the creatures kept referring to the ship's crew as "ugly bags of mostly water." I didn't know about the "ugly" part, but I was struck by the idea that we humans are not much more than walking bags of flesh filled with water and some bones. I didn't know it then, but that TV creature was right: We are mostly water. In fact, the human body is more than 65 percent water—that means we're more water than solid matter—much like the planet we live on. It's always struck me as more than an amazing coincidence that our bodies have the same ratio of water to solid matter as the surface of this incredible planet we live on.

Nothing on this planet can live without water—and that includes us. Aside from oxygen, water is the nutrient we humans need

47

most. But most of us don't give water much thought, not even when we mindlessly turn on the shower in the morning. Our lack of water awareness is extremely harmful to our health and well-being.

Water is much more important to our survival than food is. A person can live for weeks without eating but will die within days without water. Why is this? This is true because water is not something that our bodies store in any meaningful way. It is something that we constantly need to replenish or else our bodies will not be able to function.

The average adult loses about 2.5 quarts of water every single day—that's about 10 cups! And that's why health professionals are constantly exhorting us to drink 8 to 10 glasses of water a day. (Contrary to popular belief, this is not an arbitrary or unreasonably high recommendation.) In fact, I would argue that 8 to 10 glasses of water a day is barely adequate, as it replaces only the water we lose while we are at rest. It doesn't account for what we lose given a whole host of other variables, such as how much we exercise in a day, how hot the climate is, or what kind of environment we're working in (dry, overheated, etc.). So instead of thinking about 10 glasses of water a day as a stretch, know that it is simply replacing what you will lose, and go for more than that.

We lose water primarily through perspiration, respiration, and urination. Our need for water becomes stunningly clear to us when we understand that we lose water every time we simply take a breath. In fact, just the process of respiration causes us to lose 2 cups of water every single day. Without even being aware that we're sweating, we're losing an additional 2 cups a day to water that is evaporating off our skin. And each time we urinate, we're losing another cup or so of water, or roughly an additional 6 cups during a 24-hour period. Despite this rather impressive amount of water loss, few of us even come close to replacing this lost water each day. Why is this?

Much like the sorry Standard American Diet, I think we can blame our parched ways on the pace of modern life. "Modern life is like a marathon," wrote Lee Reilly in an article for *Vegetarian Times*. It is sustained activity punctuated by opportunities to drink water." Unfortunately, most of us ignore the chances to stop at life's watering stations and tank up. I love Reilly's analogy that life is like a marathon. But we're killing ourselves by not replenishing our fluids appropriately during this race that we call modern life. Think about that for a moment. Would you ever consider lacing up your running shoes and running more than 26 miles without taking a drink of water? I didn't think so. So why are most of us skipping right past those watering holes every day of our lives?

Part of the problem is that our brains have become so distracted from our bodies that we just don't heed the call when our bodies are crying out for water. In fact, most of us are already dehydrated by the time we stop to take a drink. Dehydration, clinically speaking, is when we have lost 1 to 2 percent of our weight in fluids. It can seriously affect the functioning of every part of the body, from the brain to the kidneys and the heart. According to nutrition expert Paul Stitt, author of *The Real Cause of Heart Disease,* 75 percent of Americans are constantly dehydrated, and the thirst response mechanism in most of us is so dulled that a whopping 37 percent of us mistake thirst for hunger! In short, we're so out of touch with our watery selves that we don't even notice the difference between when we need to take a drink and when we need to eat. The consequences of this distraction can be quite costly—and, when extreme, even fatal.

Mild dehydration is one of the great plagues of modern life. It slows down the body's metabolic processes and overtaxes our kidneys. Common symptoms of even mild dehydration include dry mouth, fatigue, lethargy, muscle weakness or cramps, headaches, dizziness, nausea, and forgetfulness. More-severe dehydration can cause mental confusion, asthma attacks, and sunken eyes. If your urine is a bright or dark yellow (and you're not taking a vitamin B complex supplement, which will color your urine) and has a strong smell, this is another sign that your water intake is just too low.

Extreme dehydration can have dire consequences on our health. The onset of severe dehydration while exercising can trigger heatstroke, which is characterized by an extremely high fever and the shutting down of the sweat system, which, in effect, turns off the body's thermostat. Once this happens, the internal temperature of the body can rise precipitously, which can lead to death. During severe dehydration, the heart is also forced to work harder because it has less blood available (remember, blood is mostly water) to pump through the system. The heart that is straining under these circumstances can begin to beat irregularly, and this can lead to cardiac arrest.

By taking in a minimum of just 10 cups of water a day, most of us would feel markedly better in global ways, and we would be helping to ward off some very serious illnesses, too.

Once most of my clients come clean about it, they are surprised to discover how little water they actually drink. They drink lots of sodas, coffee, and juices, and many hold the mistaken assumption that they're getting enough water from these beverages. Many of them also tell me that they just don't like drinking water, which I always find kind of perplexing but not surprising. Of course, most of us would rather bypass a beverage that is clean and naturally taste-free for a drink that comes in a pretty bottle and is loaded with sugars, chemicals, additives, and flavor enhancers that excite our brains and our tastebuds. We've become well trained to quench our thirst with these intensely flavored, often sugary beverages that the food industry markets so aggressively. Once you've become accustomed to drinking only sugary sodas and juices, water seems beyond bland by comparison.

My client Sara was having a tough time remembering to drink water throughout the day. Sara is a busy entertainment executive who works at her desk all day—and her office gets hot, as it faces south in a large office building in New York City. Sara decided to focus on water in a different way by bringing a beautiful glass water pitcher to work. She placed the pitcher on a pretty tray with a few matching glasses and filled the pitcher with fresh, cool water every day. Now when she is working for hours at a time, her eyes are drawn to the pitcher and she is reminded to continue sipping water throughout the day. Whenever someone stops by for a meeting, Sara offers them a glass of water also. Some days, she adds slices of citrus fruit, like lemons, limes, or oranges or cucumber, fresh mint, or basil.

To find out if you're taking in enough water, I urge you to take the simple water quiz on the next page.

## WHY WATER IS THE KEY TO DETOXIFING YOUR BODY

Water is, quite literally, the river on which our good health flows. Water carries nutrients to our cells, aids digestion by forming stomach secretions, flushes our bodies of wastes, and keeps our kidneys healthy. It keeps our moisture-rich organs (our skin, eyes, mouth, and nose) functioning well, it lubricates and cushions our joints, and it regulates our body temperature and our metabolism, just to name a few of its many functions.

Water also plays a crucial role in disease prevention. In a study conducted at the Centre for Human Nutrition at the University of Sheffield, England, researchers concluded that women who stay adequately hydrated reduce their risk of breast cancer by 79 percent. Another study, done at the Fred Hutchinson Cancer Research Center in Seattle, found that women who drink more than five glasses of water a day have a 45 percent reduced risk of colon cancer compared with women who drink two or fewer glasses of water a day.

Many doctors believe that proper hydration can help prevent chronic joint diseases, such as rheumatoid arthritis, because water reduces inflammation and promotes cartilage health.

Adequate water consumption can also slow the signs of aging and improve conditions such as constipation, diabetes, hypoglycemia, obesity, arthritis, kidney stones, dry skin, wrinkles, cataracts, and glaucoma.

# H₂O: The Toxic Avenger

Without enough water flowing through our systems to carry out wastes and toxins, we would literally drown in our own poisonous metabolic wastes. I don't mean to sound alarmist, but this is no exaggeration. Even slight dehydration can wear down our systems in ways that seriously compromise our overall quality of life.

Just as the liver is crucial to the digestive process, the kidneys are necessary for helping the body remove water and waste. The kidneys are a pair of small organs that are located near the spine at the small of the back. They take in about 20 percent of the body's blood each time the heart beats, cleans it of unwanted substances and then produce urine, the fluid by which these wastes are eliminated from the body. Normal-functioning kidneys also control the concentration levels of body fluids. If body fluids are too dilute, the kidneys expel excess water via urine. If body fluids are too concentrated, the kidneys excrete the excess solutes and hang on to the water. In short, the kidneys are all about balancing the fluids and electrolytes in our bodies so that our systems run smoothly.

If the kidneys don't get the water they need to perform these filtering functions, our health deteriorates rapidly.

*Electrolyte* is the scientific term for a type of salt made up of ions that are positively and negatively charged. These are the "sparks" that transfer electrical messages across cells, and this activity is what makes our bodies function. Our kidneys work to keep our electrolyte concentrations steady, since they must be replaced constantly. If they're not, dehydration can set in, which can lead to organ damage and seizures. How can we be sure that we're getting enough electrolytes? Do we need to buy specially formulated, sugar-enhanced sports drinks? Many sports physiologists actually recommend water—that's right, plain water—over the fancy sports drinks that are marketed to us. Experts have found that the difference in electrolyte content between water and sports drinks is important only to elite athletes who are competing professionally in endurance events. Since electrolytes are already plentiful in the American diet, moderate to regular exercisers don't have to worry about running out of these salty ions. Edible sea vegetables, the most nutrient-dense foods on the planet, are a great source of electrolytes as well as of minerals and trace elements.

According to Traditional Chinese Medicine, the kidneys and bladder regulate the fluids in our bodies and make up the Water Element. Our kidneys are fantastic waste removers; they get rid of the waste products from protein metabolism—uric acid, urea, and lactic acid—but they need lots of water to accomplish this.

Traditional Chinese Medicine reveres the kidneys because they distribute *qi*, or vital life energy, throughout the body. The kidneys are responsible for removing excess hormones, vitamins, minerals, and foreign toxins such as drugs, chemicals, and food additives.

## EATING FOR KIDNEY HEALTH

*Eat more:* Asparagus, bananas, celery, cucumbers, garlic, legumes, papaya, parsley, plain yogurt, potatoes, pumpkin, raw foods, seeds, soybeans, spirulina, sprouts, watercress, watermelon, whole grains

If you wish to further supplement your diet to support kidney health, you can take acidophilus (which is an active culture found in yogurt) or lecithin (which is found in soybeans and whole grains).
*Eat less:* Beet greens, meat, phosphates, potassium, rhubarb, spinach, Swiss chard
*Avoid:* Chocolate, cocoa, dairy, eggs
*Drink:* At least 10 glasses of water a day

## WATER FIGHTS FAT

Drinking water is hugely beneficial for weight loss. In fact, if you're looking for a magic bullet to get your weight loss under way, there is no better strategy than to drink 10 glasses of water a day. Here's why: Water is a natural appetite suppressor, and it helps the body metabolize fat. When the kidneys don't get enough water and can't function properly, the liver gets called upon to fill in and take on the role of eliminating toxins from our systems. Normally, one of the liver's big jobs is to metabolize stored fat into a usable form of energy. But when the liver is busy doing the kidneys' job, it's not available to metabolize stored fat. As more and more fat is stored in the body, weight loss stops.

Paradoxically, drinking lots of water is also a best remedy for water retention. The body retains water as a response to not getting enough water in the first place. Perceiving a threat, the cells cling onto the water they have, causing swelling in our hands, feet, and legs. When we drink enough water, our cells can relax and do their job—without holding on to scarce water.

Also, someone who is overweight needs to take in more water than someone who is thin. This is because the larger person has a larger metabolic load. To support this, more water is needed.

As you are losing weight, your body is going to have more toxins and waste to dispose of. Step up your water intake at this point, and you'll help your body eliminate wastes more efficiently, thereby helping your weight loss along.

## Three Stimulating Reasons to Drink More Water

If you indulge in any of the following three stimulants, you'll need extra water in your diet to counteract their dehydrating effects.

**SALT.** When you have too much salt in your system, water molecules exit your blood cells to dilute and get rid of the excess salt. This means that they are immediately lacking the water they need to function normally. These crippled cells try to carry the excess salt to your kidneys, which can become overtaxed and even shut down. The Standard American Diet is salt-heavy, and we need to counter it by drinking more water. The average American takes in about 6 to 18 grams, or 1 to 3 teaspoons, of salt daily. Your body actually needs only about 0.5 gram of salt a day for basic functions. Keep this in mind when you are working to take in enough water.

**ALCOHOL.** Your brain is 76 percent water, which explains why alcohol-induced hangovers cause headaches—alcohol is so dehydrating that it literally dries out your brain cells! And this, of course, makes your head hurt. If you're going to drink, be two-fisted and drink at least a full glass of water for every serving of alcohol you have. Better yet, make that two to one.

**CAFFEINE.** Caffeine is a diuretic, which means it prompts the kidneys to produce urine. If you drink coffee, make sure you counter the effects of the caffeine in it by drinking at least 4 ounces of water for every cup of coffee you have. Also, caffeine is a stimulant, and so it gives you an almost instant jolt of "energy." But this usually doesn't last. The next time you are feeling sluggish and reach for a cup of coffee, have two glasses of water instead and see how refreshed and energized you feel.

## WATER: THE QUALITY COUNTS

Now that you understand how important drinking water is to your health and your detox, you're probably thinking that all you have to do is turn on the tap, fill a glass, and get on with it. I wish it were that simple. Unfortunately, our nation's water supply is not as pristine as it once was, so I encourage all of you to be a little bit picky when it comes to your water. Heavy metals, pesticides, antibiotics and other drugs, disinfection by-products, radioactive particles, bacteria, and chemicals can be found in municipal water supplies in most states across the country.

Probably the most common toxin still found in water is lead. Though the use of lead paint was banned in the United States in 1978, many older homes have plumbing systems that may still contain lead parts. Lead contamination is a serious concern, especially because of the impact of lead poisoning on children's health. If a young child ingests too much lead, it can lead to learning disabilities, blood poisoning, seizures, and even death.

Mercury is another common contaminant found in water samples in many U.S. cities. In 2003, the Environmental Protection Agency (EPA) released a study showing that in 1 year, the amount of mercury detected in American rivers increased by 65 percent, which means that more than 850,000 miles of fresh water and 14 million acres of lakes are contaminated with this toxic metal.

If you suspect that your home's water may be contaminated with any of these heavy metals, you can reduce the amount by running the water for at least 30 to 60 seconds before using it. The first run of water will flush out most of the heavy metals that may have accumulated in the pipes. Or you can filter your water using one of several filtration systems I'll mention later in this chapter.

Another alarming trend is that prescription medications are being to show up in our water supply. No one yet knows what this kind of hidden "mass medicating" will do to the population, but awareness of this category of toxin is yet another reason to filter water before drinking it.

While chlorination of our nation's water supplies has been credited with all but eliminating diseases such as cholera and typhoid, chlorine is also one of the most toxic elements on the periodic chart. Long used as an ingredient in bleaching cleansers, and useful for killing germs and other microorganisms, chlorine is very dangerous in elevated quantities. Our local and state governments use chlorine to sanitize our water supplies, yet there are no guarantees that people who are sensitive to chemicals will not have an adverse reaction to this additive. The good news is that chlorine will evaporate. If you are not using a water filter, leave your water uncovered and at room temperature for at least an hour before drinking it in order to purge it of chlorine. Your skin absorbs minerals and chemicals, too, so think about putting a chlorine filter on your showerhead.

Methyl tertiary butyl ether (MTBE), a chemical additive in gasoline, has been slowly leaking from underground tanks in gasoline stations and creeping into our water tables since 1979. MTBE was believed to be the answer for oil companies who wanted to create less air pollution by making their products burn cleaner. This additive has been linked with liver and kidney problems, headaches, nose and throat problems, birth defects, dizziness, and cancer. Filtration is necessary to eliminate this substance from your water—it won't evaporate away like chlorine. To find out if your area or water table has been contaminated by MTBE, contact your local water utility for more information. Testing information and kits can be ordered from www.aquamd.com.

We all know that fluoride is put into our toothpaste in order to prevent tooth decay. But did you also know that many cities and states add fluoride to their drinking water? *Hydrofluorosilicic acid* is collected from industrial smokestack filters during the production of phosphate fertilizer and sold to cities in North America, which then add this industrial-grade source of fluoride to drinking water. This type of fluorosilicate has not been tested for safety in humans, unlike the more expensive pharmaceutical-grade sodium fluoride salt, which is what is put into toothpaste. (But even this is not known to be safe: That is why there are warnings on toothpaste that say "do not swallow.") All of this fluoride doesn't seem to be helping us much. Evidence compiled by the World Health Organization shows no advantage in levels of tooth decay in countries that use fluoridated water compared with countries that do not. But health officials do know that too much fluoride can be bad for us: It can accumulate in the bones, making them brittle and causing them to fracture, increasing the risk for osteoporosis; it can damage tooth enamel; it has been found to facilitate the absorption of heavy metals such as lead and aluminum into the blood and brain, especially in children; and it can inhibit the immune system. Flouride can even be found in bottled water and other packaged foods and beverages. The addition of fluoride to our water supply is unnecessary, because fluoride occurs naturally in the appropriate trace amounts our bodies need. My recommendation? Filter it out.

The EPA recommends that people with weakened immune systems boil their water for 1 minute before consuming it to reduce contamination levels, yet many chemicals and heavy metals actually become more concentrated in the boiling process, so I would be wary of relying on this as the sole method by which you filter water.

Filtering your own water at home is absolutely the best way to ensure its quality. The initial expense of a home filter may seem high, but in a short time the filter will pay for itself, compared with the cost of buying bottled water. Carbon-filter pitchers, reverse-osmosis filters, and ceramic filters are all available for home use and help improve a variety of contaminant issues. Showerhead filters are also available and can help to decrease the amount of toxins your body comes into contact with through the skin.

**CARBON-FILTER PITCHERS.** The most popular and least expensive filter, most are pitchers that hold a small carbon-filled filter that removes most heavy metals, chlorine, chemicals, pesticides, herbicides, insecticides, and radioactive particles from water. However, most of these filters do not remove fluoride, arsenic, viruses, some heavy metals, and nitrates. These filters are also known to breed bacteria if not changed often enough.

**CARBON/REVERSE-OSMOSIS COMBINATION FILTERS.** The initial higher cost of a reverse-osmosis filter can be well worth it, given that it will remove everything that a carbon filter does, plus MTBE, bacteria, viruses, parasites, arsenic, heavy metals, fluoride, sulfates, nitrates, radioactive particles, and asbestos. These filters can be mounted on countertops or underneath kitchen sinks and work in conjunction with your plumbing system to offer water on demand.

**CERAMIC FILTERS.** Ceramic filters eliminate bacteria, cysts, chlorine, foul taste and odor, herbicides, and pesticides. Many ceramic filters have silver baked into them, which inhibits the bacterial growth that can be a problem with standard carbon filters. These filters come in countertop versions and versions that can be mounted under the sink. They can be paired with fluoride filters if you live in a municipality that heavily fluoridates its water.

**DISTILLED WATER.** Sometimes labeled in individual bottles as "purified water," distilled water has been put through a steaming process to remove almost all impurities. However, this water is also considered to be "dead" by many health experts, as it contains no naturally occurring minerals or trace elements. For people who are intensely detoxifying for a short period of time, this water may be useful in terms of making sure that all toxins—for the short term—are eliminated. But in general, I recommend filtered water over distilled water.

## The Hidden Risks of Plastic Bottles

Convenience can be a great thing—we're lucky to have easy access to portable water sources all day in America. Bottled water can be found in gas stations, convenience stores, and most vending machines. However, there is some concern about the types of plastics being used to store this precious liquid. Plastic is made from petroleum, or oil. Exposure to the chemicals and solvents used to make plastics can cause serious health problems. It is difficult to avoid using plastics, especially if we're trying to up our water intake. But there are some precautions we can take so that we're not drinking the plastic-born toxins with our water: Avoid freezing any bottled water, as freezing leads to leaching of chemicals into the liquid. Avoid using plastic bottles for warm or hot liquids, as the heat causes a similar effect. And avoid washing and reusing your water bottles: Each time you wash them, more chemicals are released from the plastic, and you'll end up drinking more than you bargained for.

# Skin: Drench It for Good Health

Your skin is your largest detoxification organ—clean, clear skin can be a sign of good health, and blemished, blotchy skin can be a warning sign of toxicity. Now, for those teenagers out there, be aware that hormones and puberty play a part in your overall skin condition. Many toxic qualities in our bodies are carried through our circulatory systems to our skin, where they are flushed out through normal perspiration. However, your diet of food and water can be the most important factor in keeping skin glowing and vibrant. When our main blood-cleansing organs, including the kidneys, don't get enough water to function properly, the effects of this may show up on our faces or bodies: Rashes and acne can be the body's signal that harmful toxins are being ingested and are not being detoxed from our bodies. Getting enough water of good quality is another step on the road to a toxin-free body. Use water as a flushing tool— set a goal to drink enough water to replace your daily perspiration— and know that while you are supporting your kidneys, you are also protecting the health of your skin. Glowing, well-hydrated, healthy skin is like a beautiful garden—you have to water it regularly!

# How to Boost Your Water Intake

Here are the tips I share with my clients on how to get enough water in their diets.

- Drink one to two glasses of water as soon as you get up in the morning. You have been asleep for 6 to 10 hours, and that's a long time to go without any liquids. (This often helps people overcome their addictions to caffeine, as rehydrating the body and brain lead to clearer thinking and better energy.)
- Keep a beautiful pitcher of filtered water near your work space so that you are constantly reminded to drink during the day. Fill up the pitcher with the amount of water you want to consume in the day.
- Drink a glass of water before exercise.
- During exercise, drink about 8 ounces of fluid every 15 to 20 minutes.

- Avoid drinks with caffeine or alcohol, which have a dehydrating effect.

- Never restrict the amount of water you crave during regular exercise.

- Always make fluids a part of your exercise routine.

- Bottles, bottles everywhere! Keep bottles of water in your car, at the office, or around your work areas. One client of mine bought a whole case and kept it in the trunk of her car!

- To reduce the amount of chlorine in your drinking water if you aren't using a filter, try this simple tip: Allow drinking water to stand at room temperature for an hour or more, which will allow most of the chlorine to evaporate out of the water.

- Drink at least one glass of room-temperature water with every meal.

## KITCHEN PREP: JUNKING THE JUNK

This first week of your detox diet is a time of preparation and planning. In order to prepare your life, and specifically your kitchen, for a new way of preparing and eating food, you need to detox those shelves, drawers, and cabinets. Cleaning out toxic foods from the hidden corners and shelves of your kitchen will help to silence the irresistible yet toxic voices that have grown so familiar to you. Junking the junk food will unclutter your larder, so you can stay calm and focused on the goal at hand: your detox. The best way to do this is to become a "food detective," as my mentor Joshua would say. Get to know what the snacks and treats you relied on in the past are really made of by reading the ingredient labels. Toss out anything that is full of sugar, chemicals, preservatives, and other toxic ingredients that you no longer want mucking up your body. Use the following list of common food additives, which is from the Center for Science in the Public Interest (www.cspinet.org), as a guide while you remove any suspect food products from your life.

**BLUE 1.** Artificial coloring found in beverages, candy, and baked goods. Insufficiently studied; linked with some cancers.

**BLUE 2.** Artificial coloring found in pet food, beverages, and candy. Possibly linked with brain tumors in animal studies.

**RED 3.** Artificial coloring found in fruit cocktail cherries, candies, and baked goods. Evidence of a link with thyroid tumors.

**YELLOW 6.** Artificial coloring found in beverages, sausages, baked goods, candy, and gelatin. Linked with tumors and allergic reactions.

**ACESULFAME-K.** Artificial sweetener found in baked goods, chewing gum, soft drinks, and gelatin desserts. Animal studies have suggested that the additive might cause cancer and affect thyroid function.

**HYDROGENATED AND PARTIALLY HYDROGENATED VEGETABLE OILS.** Found in shortenings, margarines, crackers, fried restaurant foods, and baked goods. Contain *trans fat*, which leads to heart disease.

**POTASSIUM BROMATE.** A flour improver used in processed breads and rolls. Bromates cause cancer in animals.

**PROPYL GALLATE.** An antioxidant preservative found in vegetable oils, meat products, processed potato products, chewing gum, and some chicken soups. Used to stop the spoilage of fats, it has been suggested that this additive may cause cancer.

**SACCHARIN.** Artificial sweetener found in diet drinks and products, also known as Sweet 'N Low. Strongly linked with causing cancer.

**SODIUM NITRATE AND SODIUM NITRITE.** Preservative, coloring, and flavoring used in processed meats, bacon, and smoked fish. Can cause formation of carcinogenic chemicals in foods.

Now that your kitchen has been detoxed and you've begun to pump up your water intake, it is time to think about the "larger picture" aspects of your detox. To that end, spend a little time with yourself. Begin to get to know what you really want your diet—and your life—to look like.

## STRESS LESSEN
### Herbal Baths

Now that water is becoming more important in your daily life and you've begun your detox, reward yourself with one of the easiest, most enjoyable stress reducers available: Take a hot bath! Let yourself relax into a simple scented bath for a calming spa treatment at home.

*For each bath, follow these directions:* Combine all ingredients in a piece of cheesecloth or in the toe of an old pair of panty hose. Tie up the open end with a piece of string, and place this pouch in the tub before you run your bath. As the tub fills with water, the soothing scents and healing properties of these sachets will be released. Sit back and enjoy!

For a *refreshing* bath, try some of the following herbs: bay leaves, basil, rosemary, mint, pine leaves, or thyme.

For a *relaxing* bath, try one or any combination of these herbs: catnip, chamomile, jasmine, or lavender.

For a *cleansing* bath, use the following herbs singly or together: borage, fennel, lemon balm, rose petals, and sage.

Or for an invigorating and exfoliating salt scrub:

For a *skin-softening* bath, combine the following in a bowl, stand in the bathwater, and rub the mixture into your skin for a few moments. Relax in the tub and gently wash the mixture off of your skin: 1 cup plain oatmeal, ½ cup salt, 10 drops lavender oil, and 1 cup water.

Finally, for those days when your body is just plain achy:

For *sore muscles,* soak ½ cup of fresh rosemary in a quart of hot water for 10 minutes, then add the strained infusion to your bath. Soak in this scented water for relaxing relief.

## MENTAL DETOX

### Map Your Detox

Making the commitment to detox your diet and your life is a profound decision. And for each of us, the reasons we're detoxing are unique. To better understand your own motivation, desires, and needs, spend some time this first week thinking about why you've decided to detox and what benefits you hope to gain from it. Look at your current state of health as well as the current state of your relationships, and think about your overall life goals. No one begins a journey without a map, so take this week as a chance to create your own detox road map.

**Exercise:** Sit down with a blank sheet of paper and a pen or pencil. Before you begin writing, look at your body, beginning with looking at your face in a mirror. What do you see? Do you look tired? Pale? Bloated? Do you have blemishes, a rash, or some other skin eruption? Record whatever it is you observe about your face. And be specific: Write about your hair, your skin, your eyes, your tongue, and your teeth. Also write down how you feel. Now move on down your body. Are you happy with the overall weight and shape of your body? Does it feel muscular or lumpy? Does it feel strong or weak and shaky? How about the skin on your arms—is it bumpy or smooth? Moving to your middle, how do your internal organs feel? Are your liver and kidneys functioning well? Further down, are your legs strong and lean? Are your knees pain-free? Do you have spider veins in your calves? What about your feet? Are your toes and toenails healthy?

Don't just look at what's wrong with your body: Write about what you like, too. Are your ears pointy in a way that you find cute? Do you have a funny-shaped pinky toe? Do you pride yourself on your lovely legs? Really take the chance to explore your body, inside and out, and to get a sense of what pleases you and what you'd like to change. It is important to have a strong understanding of where you stand today, in terms of your body image and your level of satisfaction with how your body functions. Take note of the beautiful parts as well as the parts that you would like to heal, change, or improve.

After getting a really good mental image of where you are, you can begin to picture what you want to see for yourself in the future. How do you want to feel in the morning when you wake up? What kinds of activities would you like to participate in? What changes would you like to see in your body? Do you want your mood to improve? Do you want to have less stress in your life? Do you wish to lose weight? Do you want to eat in a better way?

Writing out what we have stored in our brains accomplishes two things: It tells us where we are, and it helps us to map out where we want to go. Once you've made your goals concrete, you will be empowered to tackle your detox in ways that will truly help you reach your goals.

# CHAPTER 5

# How Sweet It Isn't

## Week 2: Rethinking Our Love Affair with Sugar
## Nutritional Issue: Sugar

Sugar is more than just a treat in this country. It has become a staple of the Standard American Diet. It is our favorite stimulant, flavor enhancer, and emotional crutch. (I have been known to use it as a boyfriend substitute.) But just 100 years ago, white cane sugar was really hard to come by: It was expensive, and it was considered a luxury item. Today, we simply can't get away from it. Sugar is added to almost every food that's stocked on the shelves of our grocery stores. From breakfast cereals and bread to snack foods and condiments, sugar is everywhere and in everything. This might seem like a good thing, since we can't seem to get enough of it! (Maybe that's why candy bars are always shelved at hand level, right in front of the cash register.)

Sugar is a carbohydrate, and we all need carbohydrates to survive—that's just a fact of living as a human being. We need them for the energy they supply to our bodies and brains. But there are good carbohydrates and bad carbohydrates, and most of us have no idea what the difference is. The kind of carbohydrates our bodies need are found mostly in plant foods, such as vegetables, fruits, beans, and grains. They are what I like to call whole carbohydrates and are most often referred to as complex carbohydrates. But we've become addicted to getting our carbs from processed foods that are loaded with additives like sugar and other sweeteners, and these are called refined carbohydrates. A recent USDA survey shows that the average American is eating and drinking about 20 teaspoons of sugar a day—that's twice the highest amount recommended by the FDA, which urges us to take in no more than 10 teaspoons a day. But how on earth can any of us do this if a single 12-ounce can of Coke has 10 teaspoons of sugar in it?

Recent reports in the media have stated that Americans have been eating less white refined sugar in the past 2 decades, down to 63.2 pounds per person per year in 2002. *That's still a lot of sugar!* This reduction in cane sugar consumption doesn't mean we're eating less sugar—now we're just getting it in another form. In the early 1980s, food companies began to use a form of sugar known as *high fructose corn syrup*, or HFCS, in their products. The reason? HFCS is significantly cheaper than cane sugar and saves the food industry tens, if not hundreds, of millions of dollars a year. USDA studies show an increase in consumption of HFCS by 250 percent over the last 15 years. Some studies show that the average American kid consumes up to 20 percent of his daily calories from HFCS alone. In the early 1960s, the average American consumed no HFCS. By 2002, the average American was consuming 62.8 pounds of HFCS a year! In less than one generation, we've become hooked on this dangerous druglike sweetener that effectively has doubled our intake of sugar additives.

Why is this corn-derived sweetener so ubiquitous and so inexpensive? It's a matter of politics. The federal government began offering subsidies to corn growers in the 1970s. This created a huge amount of dirt-cheap corn that was turned into a sweetener that is much cheaper than sugar. And if it is cheaper, it is what the food giants want.

HFCS is so cheap to produce that it has replaced cane sugar in almost every processed food we eat: sodas, juices, candies, pasta sauces, ketchup, cookies, syrups, yogurts, soups, salad dressings, breakfast cereals—even baby formula. These cheap calories are making us fat and sick. Sugars like HFCS have become so common in our food that in order to avoid them, we must truly become "food detectives" and be able to recognize when they and other empty, toxic substances are hidden on food labels.

In the early 1980s, when HFCS became commonplace in food products, a once-stable obesity level in this country began to spike, and it has been soaring ever since. How can there not be a connection?

## What's So Sweet about Eliminating Sugar from Your Diet?

Why is eliminating refined carbohydrates and sugars from your diet crucial to detoxing your body? First, there is the nutritional nature—or lack thereof—of refined carbohydrates. These foods exist in a "nutrient vacuum," meaning that most refined carbs, such as sugar, white rice, white pasta, cereals, and bread products, pretty much contain only one thing: too much refined carbohydrate. These foods are low in fiber and have been stripped of most of their nutrients—that's why so many of these products are vitamin and mineral fortified: It's the food industry's way of trying to replace what they've taken away.

Second, because these foods are lacking in vital nutrients, they're processed in the body quickly as carbs, which are converted into sugar to provide us with energy. With carbs that are high in glucose, like cane sugar, the body may experience a quick sugar high that sends its metabolic systems into overdrive. Once the sugar high wears off (our blood sugar plummets), we're left feeling hungry all over again. So we repeat this vicious cycle of eating empty foods (thereby starving our bodies of essential nutrition) that spike our sugar production, we crash, and we do it all again—without ever being aware that this is what we're doing to ourselves. Our bodies, mind you, hate this way of eating. There is simply no chance for our bodies to achieve any sort of nutritional or metabolic balance when we eat this way.

HFCS, however, appears to affect our bodies differently than sugars that convert right to glucose, behaving more like fat than sugar when it hits our bloodstreams. With fructose, there is no spike in blood sugar, and there is also no signaling to our bodies that we've been adequately fed. This is one of the potentially scary attributes of foods laced with HFCS, and it has researchers very concerned. Since HFCS doesn't appear to signal to our bodies that we've taken in calories, we tend to eat more foods laden with these than we should. In essence, when we eat foods high in HFCS, our bodies are essentially tricked into wanting to eat more, and at the same time, our bodies are processing this sugar in ways that prompt them to store more fat. This is part of the reason many experts believe our rising consumption of HFCS is a major contributor to the current obesity crisis.

Simply put, our bodies just don't know what to do with this stuff when it is consumed in the outrageous quantities found in the Standard American Diet. Reducing or eliminating your intake of sugars and sweeteners will be a huge step toward losing weight, easing the stress put on your liver, and detoxing your body.

## THE EFFECTS OF "SUGAR" ON THE HUMAN MIND AND BODY

Sugar has a druglike effect on us, because it releases opiates in the brain. The neurotransmitter serotonin is released when we eat sugar, giving us a happy, content feeling. Those "happy sensors" in our brains light up when we eat sugar, and the more of it we eat, the more we want. Human beings are born with two taste preferences—an attraction to sweet and an aversion for bitter. In his book *Breaking the Food Seduction,* Neal Barnard, M.D., writes about an amazing experiment performed at the University of Massachusetts at Amherst involving sugar's effect on babies:

> "Here is how to magnetize a baby: Start with a calm infant of 9 to 12 weeks of age. Sit face to face, about 15 inches apart. Dip a pacifier into sugar water (made by stirring a teaspoon of sugar into a cup of water) and put the pacifier in the baby's mouth. If it falls out, dip it in again and put it

back. Keep it there for 3½ minutes while maintaining consistent eye contact. That's all it takes. You can then leave the room. When you return, you will find that the baby will look at you, smile, gurgle, and maybe even throw you a coy expression. He or she will follow you with his or her eyes and clearly prefer you over other people. *What you have done is register your face in the baby's memory and connect that image with a sensation in the baby's pleasure circuitry, triggered by sugar.*"

Once a baby is hooked on sugar, it is downhill—literally—from there. In the last 5 years, three major studies on aging looked at the oldest of the old—the centenarians. While people who live to be 100 or older are becoming less rare, researchers wanted to know one thing: How did these people manage to live so long? Old fogies from around the world were questioned, analyzed, and tested, and one common theme kept reappearing: They all had low blood sugar levels for their age, and they all had low insulin levels. In short, they had eaten diets that were rich in complex carbohydrates and short on unnecessary sugars. Basically, their bodies hadn't been worn out by a constant stream of sugars that needed to be processed, detoxified, and eliminated. They had eaten in ways that kept them youthful!

The pancreas pumps out insulin to escort sugar through the blood to our tissues and muscles. If the insulin can't do its job properly, our blood sugar levels become elevated and we can run into serious problems. The more sugar you eat, the more insulin your pancreas has to produce, and the more resistant your cells become to the effects of that insulin. But your pancreas can't keep up with this heightened demand for insulin for long. When this little organ finally starts to slow down, or your resistance gets too high, your blood sugar goes up to dangerous levels, and diabetes kicks in. The bottom line is that the less refined sugar you consume, the less stress your body has to deal with, and the less likely you'll be to ever develop the serious disease of type 2 diabetes.

Insulin has other important jobs that we don't give it credit for. Insulin stores magnesium, an important mineral used by our bodies to relax our muscles and blood vessels. Our cells become insulin resistant because they're trying to protect themselves from the toxic effects of too much insulin. If your cells become insulin resistant, you can't store magnesium and it is lost through urination. The same thing happens with calcium. High levels of insulin cause your body to lose calcium, even if you're taking supplements. When your insulin goes up after a sugar binge, you lose calcium and magnesium, and your cells become even more insulin resistant. High levels of insulin affect the nervous system in a serious way, too. When our bodies become imbalanced and unable to utilize insulin properly, we head into toxic terrain and risk a host of health problems. Getting your insulin under control is *that* important.

Insulin is also involved in fat metabolism. If you are overconsuming calories from sugar, your body will produce more and more insulin in an effort to use this sugar energy. But if it cannot use this energy, your body will store it as fat, and a vicious insulin-resistance cycle is begun. As your body becomes more and more insulin resistant, your weight will go up and up. So while your fat cells are becoming more resistant, you store more fat. Now you have more fat, your blood sugar problems are causing you to produce and store more fat, and things are going from bad to worse. That extra insulin floating around in your bloodstream causes plaque to build up in your arteries, too, and this can lead to cardiovascular disease.

Now that you know all this, doesn't cutting sugar from your diet sound like a good idea? But I'll be the first to admit that cutting sugar from your diet is no easy task. We have become so sugar-dependent that giving it up is just as hard as giving up any drug.

## KICKING SUGAR OUT OF THE HOUSE

For many sugar addicts, the hardest part of kicking the habit is resisting the cookies or the pint of ice cream that calls out from the kitchen. Believe me, I've been there too. The best way to avoid falling off the sugar-free wagon is to get rid of all the sugars that may be lurking in your cupboards and refrigerator. Use this list of common names for added sugars and artificial sweeteners and see if there is sugar lurking around in places you would never suspect. Go ahead and take the plunge: Throw away the sugar that is polluting your life.

- Aspartame
- Corn syrup
- Dextrose
- Evaporated cane juice
- Fructose
- Fruit juice concentrate
- Glucose
- Golden syrup
- High fructose corn syrup
- Honey
- Invert sugar
- Lactose
- Malt
- Malt extract
- Maltitol
- Maltose
- Mannitol
- Maple syrup
- Molasses
- Rice extract
- Saccharin
- Sorbitol
- Sucrose
- Xylitol

## ARE YOU ON THE "SUGAR-CYCLE ROLLER COASTER?"

Sugar isn't always the problem—for many of us, it's the answer: the answer to our sorrows, our lack of energy, and our boredom. How does sugar become such an important part of our lives? For many of us, it starts in childhood. We were rewarded with sweets when we accomplished something deemed worthy, offered candy when we were feeling bad or sick, and showered with sugary treats when loved ones came to visit. These special events soon melted into everyday bowls of sweetened cereals, after-school snacks, and post-dinner desserts. Sugar, once truly a treat, has become the backbone of the Standard American Diet.

By the end of a day that typically includes muffins, sodas, sweetened coffee, southern-style "sweet tea," candy, cakes, or cookies, our bodies have been through several loop-de-loops on the sugar roller coaster. We use sugar to wake up in the morning. Then we eat more sugar after lunch to get us through the postlunch energy crash. After dinner we're run-down and exhausted, so we reach for a bowl of ice cream to make us feel comfortable, happy, and rewarded for a hard day's work. But in reality, each of these sugar binges is a fix following the crash we experienced after the last sugar binge.

Without most of us knowing it, we are addicted and we're nowhere near getting off that roller coaster.

Morgan experienced serious withdrawal symptoms when he ended his McBinge. Headaches, cramping, and chills plagued him for 3 days. These symptoms are side effects that might occur when you decide to eliminate sugar, but they will lessen and go away quickly. Perhaps you have been continuing to ride the roller coaster because you felt these symptoms coming on and you turned to sugar to make them retreat. Faced with feeling fatigue or pain—even for a short while—most of us would reach for what we know will relieve our suffering. But suppressing these symptoms with sugar won't solve the real problem, which is actually the sugar itself.

## THE EMOTIONAL REALM OF SUGAR ADDICTION

Remember, when we talk about detoxification, we are talking about the whole body—the organs, brain, spirit, and emotions included. During Morgan's immersion into the fast-food culture, he experienced some serious emotional issues that had never affected him before. He had mood swings, felt depressed, and often felt a general feeling of sadness. I was amazed to see his overall personality change so quickly. What was happening to him? It was disturbing and scary to watch the person I loved the most quickly fall apart. One major cause of his personality change was the amount of sugar he was eating and the emotional side effects it produced. Your body becomes overstressed and tired from too much sugar. The connection between your emotions and the exhaustion your organs and body are feeling is undeniable. But most of us have lost touch with the connection between what we eat and how we feel.

I often hear from my clients about cravings for salt and sugar. Sometimes these cravings are what our bodies need, and sometimes these cravings represent our addiction to the effect these foods have on our brain chemistry. When our mood goes from crabby and down to happy and relaxed after a treat, our bodies and brains remember that the next time stress rolls around. Carbohydrates, especially refined sugars, prompt the release in our brains of serotonin, a neurotransmitter associated with feeling calm and relaxed. In our antidepressant, pill-popping culture, perhaps we're medicating ourselves for mental and emotional problems that could be greatly improved by simply changing our diets and eliminating sugar. By feeding our fears with sugar, we are able to ignore the painful feelings that surround our lives. Perhaps exploring these emotions and thoughts would serve us better than stuffing the pain down with another package of cookies.

Do you crave sweets on a daily basis? Don't worry, you're not alone. This modern American life of ours has created a population of serious sugar fiends. We use sugar to wake up in the morning, to treat ourselves at the end of a hard day, to perk us up in the middle of the afternoon. We turn to sugar when we're lonely, when we're tired, afraid, angry, or depressed. We even use it to soothe the hurt feelings and the skinned knees of our kids. Our constant striving for perfection sets us up for daily failures that take a toll on our self-esteem and that we medicate quite effectively with sugar. In short, sugar has become the cure to our never-ending search for the ever-elusive "sweet life."

When clients of mine are trying to stop eating sugar, they often encounter the real problem of facing their addictions. Instead of going easy on themselves through this tough transition, I see them work only harder and suffer and sacrifice more. When this happens, I encourage my clients to take a step back, observe what they are feeling, and simply stay with that. Being able to look at the emotional issue that underlies our sugar addiction is a brave endeavor. Sitting alone on your couch again on a Saturday night is a lonely prospect, so it only makes sense that you would turn to your favorite men, Ben and Jerry, to comfort you. What my clients learn is that they no longer have to cope by using sugar, that they can address their emotional issues head-on, and that they can finally kiss Ben and Jerry goodbye.

But it's not easy. We use words like "sugar," "honey," "sweetie pie," and "muffin" to describe our loved ones, so why wouldn't we reach for a sweet treat when we're depressed or anxious—we are, after all, trying to make ourselves feel better. Substituting food for love can have unpleasant side effects, though: We risk piling problems such as weight gain, blood sugar problems, and emotional

## SUGAR QUIZ

Use these questions to explore your own relationship with sugar. Some of these questions may seem unrelated to that relationship, but I would argue that these are the questions that are worth looking at the most. There is a huge emotional/psychological component to our sugar addiction that most of us are unaware of. By beginning to connect the dots between the areas in our lives that need work and when we eat sugar, we may find our way to truly changing our lives and not just our diets. Again, I encourage you to keep some paper or a journal handy to write down your thoughts.

- Do you crave sweet treats on a daily basis?
- Do you drink regular and/or diet sodas often?
- Is chocolate or ice cream the answer to your sorrows?
- Do you reward yourself with candy or pastries?
- Is your day complete only with a sugary dessert at the end of it?
- Do you drink two or more alcoholic beverages a day, 5 or more days a week?
- Do you treat yourself with "bad" foods in secret, away from others?
- Do you eat with people, now or in the past, who judge your food choices?
- What areas of your life are keeping you from feeling happy (career, relationships, physical ailments, home environment, creativity, spiritual practice)?
- Do you trust or fear life's processes?
- How would you rate your emotional life on a scale of 1 to 10? (10 being amazingly good)
- Do you have nourishing, positive, intimate relationships with others?
- How is your relationship with yourself? Are you searching for perfection?

issues like depression on top of what is already going untreated in us. Taking away sugar—the most delicious emotional crutch in the world—allows us to get to the root of our problems and detox our emotional lives, too.

Erin lives in southern California and has tried numerous experiments with food to try to put an end to her mood and energy swings. Thinking that sugar was a problem, she eliminated all sugars for 1 month to see how she would feel. At the end of the month, she was more energetic and less moody, and she had conquered her sugar cravings. Thinking the worst was over, Erin decided to have an ice cream cone as a reward. After only two bites, she couldn't eat any more—it was too sweet! Her body no longer recognized sugar as being desirable. Even though Erin had lived with a sugar addiction for most of her life, after just 1 month she was able to break the hold this taste had on her body and brain. All it took was a little time and some patience!

## HOW TO RECOGNIZE SUGAR ON A FOOD LABEL

Most of us are unaware of the amount of sugar in the foods we buy. You can help yourself stop the flow of sugar into your home by making a few adjustments at the point of purchase: Become a food detective and read your labels before you put foods into your supermarket cart. If your old favorite doesn't meet your new, healthier standards, find another product that does. Don't be afraid to try new things: There are lots of options out there, and not just in traditional supermarkets. Terrific natural and organic food stores are popping up all over the country.

Whole grain products are high in complex carbohydrates and minerals. Fruits contain naturally occurring simple sugars but also provide us with water and fiber, which makes them a good choice for detoxification. Refined breads, cereals, snack foods, candy, and soda, on the other hand, usually contain lots of added sugar.

Try some of these tips when reading labels.

- Be aware that the first ingredient listed on a label is the largest ingredient in the product.

- Be wary of products that contain multiple forms of sugar and sweeteners. Barley malt, beet sugar, brown sugar, buttered syrup, caramel, carob syrup, corn syrup, date sugar, dehydrated cane juice, dextrose, Florida crystals, glucose, golden syrup, high fructose corn syrup, sorbitol, sorghum syrup, sugar, turbinado, xylitol, and anything ending in -os may all be listed separately, but these are all sugar and can constitute a big portion of the food.

- Look out for long lists of ingredients on a seemingly simple food product. This may point to lots of added sugar and chemical preservatives that you are now trying to avoid.

- Avoid the artificial sweeteners aspartame and saccharin.

- "Fat-free" foods might seem like a healthy choice, but they are usually full of sugar.

- Alcohol, which is loaded with sugar, is devoid of nutrients, so it is not required to carry a nutritional label.

- "Sugar free" means that the product contains less than ½ gram of sugar per serving.

- "Reduced sugar" means that the product contains 25 percent less sugar per serving than the original food product.

- The words "made with real fruit" can be sorely misleading— the law doesn't require the label to tell *how much* real fruit is actually in the food. This claim is often misused on labels on kids' snacks. That yogurt may have one or two pieces of apple floating around in it, but it's really made mostly of sugar.

- Fruit "drinks" are a regular culprit in the sugar wars. These sweet beverages may contain little or no real fruit juice. "Drink" in the name on the label is a big warning sign that this beverage is not 100 percent juice. Added sugar and water make up most fruit drinks. Choose fruit juices that are listed as "100 percent fruit juice."

## TOO MUCH OF A GOOD THING: SUGAR AND INTESTINAL PROBLEMS

Eating sugary snacks for breakfast or an afternoon pick-me-up is common for many of us. Tired after lunch? Have a coffee and a cookie. The sugar and caffeine do wake us up for a little while, but then they lead us to further exhaustion and other health problems. Sugar increases bacterial growth and fermentation activity in the intestines. The friendly bacteria in your intestines can easily be weakened by a diet full of sugar, refined foods, acidic coffee, too much animal protein, and stress. When these "good" bacteria, such as *lactobacilli,* are damaged, they can't do their job of metabolizing sugar properly. This allows the "bad" bacteria to overgrow—all of us have *Candida albicans* in our guts, but a diet high in refined carbohydrates can contribute to their rapid overgrowth.

Some women suffer from yeast infections when their intestinal flora is unbalanced. Men also suffer from this condition, known as *candidiasis* and the infection can spread throughout the body as it travels through the bloodstream and affects the organs. Symptoms are wide-ranging, but the most common include abdominal pain, headaches, constipation, bad breath, rectal itching, mood swings, memory loss, fatigue, depression, acne, sinus problems, PMS, vaginitis, irritable bowel syndrome (IBS), bladder infections, and thrush. Why should we worry about candidiasis? After all, it's only a little single-celled fungus. This little fungus releases toxins that can further weaken your immune system, leading to other problems. To keep this nasty critter from getting out of hand, integrate the following:

- Avoid all dietary sugar (including honey, maple syrup, and sugar), alcohol, cheese, dried fruit (which has a high sugar content), peanuts, baked goods, raw mushrooms, sprouts, vinegars, gluten-containing grains (wheat, oats, spelt, rye, and barley), and all food allergens, as these can make the candida worse.

- If you're taking antibiotics, which kill off all bacteria, not just the harmful ones, be sure to take an acidophilus or bifidus supplement to revive your gut's "good" bacteria.

- To avoid candida overgrowth, eat more "cultured" or "fermented" foods, such as organic plain yogurt, miso, naturally fermented sauerkraut, and olives, which provide important bacteria and enzymes that are beneficial to digestion.

- Eat more fresh garlic, which inhibits the candida fungus.

- A link has been made between high levels of mercury in the body and candida overgrowth. Consider having a hair or urine test done to determine if you have mercury toxicity, especially if you have silver mercury fillings.

- Avoid conventionally produced animal products such as meats, chicken, and dairy as they may contain antibiotics. Choose organically raised and produced animal products only, which are not raised on antibiotics.

## KICK THE CAN: TOO MUCH SUGAR IN COLAS

A main source of the precipitous rise in sugar consumption in this country is our reliance on soft drinks. Soft-drink consumption has soared in recent years: Consumption by adults climbed 61 percent, and consumption by adolescents climbed by more than 100 percent between 1977 and 1997.

Water, milk, juice, coffee, and tea are being replaced by sugar-filled colas, which also contain other toxic ingredients that harm us in unseen ways. For example, the chemical phosphoric acid, which is found in sodas, is known to interfere with the body's ability to absorb and maintain calcium levels. This can lead to a general softening of the teeth and bones and the more serious and debilitating condition of osteoporosis. Remember the story about the science fair project where a nail left in a glass of cola dissolves away? Imagine what your bones must be feeling. The additional caffeine contained in many sodas also causes jitters, insomnia, high cholesterol, and high blood pressure, and it also contributes to possible vitamin and mineral depletion.

Diet colas may seem like a better choice for those of us concerned with our sugar intakes, but there are real dangers in swapping sugar for artificial sweeteners. The artificial sweetener aspartame is a chemical compound (phenylalanine and aspartic acid) created from petrochemicals. NutraSweet, a brand name of aspartame, is unstable in the human body—it breaks down above 85°F not only into its constituent amino acids but into methanol, which can then break down into formaldehyde. Formaldehyde which is highly toxic and a known carcinogen.

Symptoms of aspartame overload or sensitivity are wide-ranging and dangerous—complaints regarding aspartame make up 80 to 85 percent of food complaints registered with the FDA. Aspartame intoxication symptoms can manifest as insomnia, nausea, headaches, blurred vision, seizures, rashes, anxiety attacks, mood changes, loss of energy, muscle and joint pain, hearing loss, loss of limb control, menstrual cramps, and heart attack–like symptoms. Artificial sweeteners have actually been found inside of brain tumors that have been removed and examined by scientists.

Amazingly, the American Cancer Society confirmed in a report that users of artificial sweeteners, including aspartame, actually gained more weight than those who didn't use the products, further undermining the supposed "purpose" of these chemicals in our foods and drinks. As you know, when we consume a significant amount of carbohydrates, the level of serotonin in our brains rises, making us feel happy, calm, and relaxed. Aspartame has a different effect on the brain when paired with carbohydrates: The brain ceases to produce serotonin, so that "I've had enough" feeling never happens. This may cause us to eat more food, and we tend to turn to the foods we know, so we pick up something else that contains aspartame, thinking it is better for our "diets." But we're not the only ones getting "fat" from this additive: In the 1990s, Monsanto made more than $900 million a year from its NutraSweet division alone—that's pretty sweet.

Sugar's journey through our bodies is complex, but it's a quick way to throw off your natural balance. When you eat sugar, it moves from your stomach directly into your blood. Your pancreas is signaled by your brain to release insulin, which acts as a little escort to move the sugar out of your blood and into your tissues and muscles. Any problems that develop with insulin resistance, overproduction, or underproduction can manifest as disease and toxicity. When the pancreas is overtaxed because we're constantly eating refined sugar, production of insulin and other hormones such as somatostatin, gastrin, and glucagons is thrown off.

Traditional Chinese Medicine has long associated an overconsumption of "sweet" with kidney, spleen, and pancreas damage. Too much sugar simply overtaxes these vital organs. Sugar also depresses the immune system, leaving us less able to deal with illness and disease. Symptoms associated with too many refined carbohydrates in your diet and in your body are excess weight, fatigue, excessive sleepiness, depression, brain fog, bloating, low blood sugar, high blood pressure, and high triglyceride levels.

## THE BENEFITS OF NATURAL SWEETENERS

Natural sweeteners are preferable to refined sugar and high fructose corn syrup because they have less of a negative impact on our bodies. Transitioning to sweeteners such as agave nectar, brown rice syrup, and date sugar can ease the daily stress that our sweet diets put on our bodies. Because these sweeteners are less processed, they do not have as dramatic an effect on blood sugar levels as the more highly refined sugar, and so they tax the body less. Not only do natural sweeteners cause less of a spike in the body's blood sugar levels, but they also still contain key nutrients that help the body with sugar metabolism. As a result, these natural sweeteners can be very helpful for balancing energy and blood sugar concerns while satisfying the sweet tooth.

*Agave nectar* is a natural liquid derived from the agave cactus. It does not contain processing chemicals and is safe for children. Agave absorbs slowly into the body, decreasing the highs and lows associated with sucrose intake as its glycemic index is very low. It is appropriate for people with diabetes, people who have carbohydrate-intolerant hypoglycemia, and those who are sensitive to sugar and corn syrup. Agave nectar is useful for baking and cooking; replace 1 cup of sugar with ¾ cup of agave nectar. Reduce recipe liquids by ⅓ and oven temperature by 25°F.

*Barley malt syrup* is, like rice syrup, mostly maltose and therefore has a mild effect on blood sugar levels. Be aware that some brands of barley malt can be blended with corn. Since it does contain gluten, barley malt syrup should be avoided by people with celiac disease.

*Date sugar* is made from grinding up pitted, dehydrated dates. About 65 percent fructose and sucrose, it is more natural and unrefined than most sweeteners. It contains the same nutrients as dried dates and works great as a replacement for white cane sugar in baking.

*Florida crystals* is a refined sugar made without the use of additives, preservatives, or animal by-products. Use sparingly.

*Fruit juice concentrates* (such as peach, grape, pear, and apple) are frozen products made by cooking down juices to produce a sweeter, more concentrated product.

*Honey* can be 25 to 60 percent sweeter than sugar due to its high fructose content. There is no industry standard for

---

# A Sweet Transition

Transitioning away from refined sugar to natural and unrefined sweeteners is a great way to satisfy your sweet urges. Cooking and preparing foods with natural sweeteners is easy, and by using the chart below, you can experiment with the wide variety of tastes and levels of sweetness available.

| NATURAL SWEETENER | EQUIVALENT TO REPLACE ½ CUP OF WHITE OR BROWN SUGAR |
|---|---|
| Agave nectar**** | ⅓ cup |
| Barley malt syrup | 1½ cups |
| Brown rice syrup*** | 1½ cups |
| Date sugar | 1 cup |
| Florida crystals | ½ cup |
| Fruit juice concentrate | ½ cup |
| Honey* | ⅓ cup |
| Maple crystals | ½ cup |
| Maple syrup | ½ cup |
| Molasses** | ⅔ cup |
| Sucanat | ½ cup |

### NOTES
■ When using liquid sweeteners as substitutes for dry, reduce or eliminate other liquid ingredients (such as water and milk) in the original recipe, and increase flour a small amount at a time, to taste.

measuring this, as each type of honey varies from the next.

*Maple crystals* are nearly 100 percent sucrose. They are a refined, powdered version of maple syrup.

*Maple syrup* is nearly 65 percent sucrose as opposed to white sugar, which is 99 percent. Forty gallons of sap are needed to produce 1 gallon of syrup.

*Molasses* is a strongly flavored, thick dark-brown syrup ob-

■ For breads, muffins, and pies, fruit juice concentrates and other liquid sweeteners such as maple syrup work well.

■ Some original recipes list no liquids, and using a dry, granulated substitute such as Sucanat, date sugar, or maple crystals will work well. To most closely copy a recipe for cakes, cupcakes, and other traditional pastries, maple crystals and Sucanat work best.

■ Baked goods and sweets made with natural sweetener substitutions are more subtle in their sweetness than are traditional goods made with refined white or brown sugar.

■ For more flavor, try adding dried fruit to muffins, scones, and cookies. Add spices such as cinnamon, cloves, and nutmeg to other baked goods to increase aroma and flavor.

*Honey: Reduce another liquid in the recipe by 2 tablespoons and add $1/4$ teaspoon baking soda per cup of honey. Reduce oven temperature by 25°F and increase baking time as necessary. Substituting honey for sugar alters the flavor and tends to make baked goods moister, chewier, and darker.

**Molasses: When substituting molasses for sugar, add $1/2$ teaspoon of baking powder for each $1/2$ cup of molasses. Reduce another liquid in the recipe by 2 tablespoons and reduce the oven temperature by 25°F. Molasses imparts a distinctive flavor and tends to make moister, chewier, and darker baked goods.

***Rice syrup: Reduce another liquid in the recipe by $1/4$ cup and add $1/4$ cup extra flour.

****Agave nectar: Replace 1 cup sugar with $3/4$ cup of agave nectar. Reduce other recipe liquids by $1/3$ and reduce oven temperature by 25°F.

tained from the refining of sugar cane. Fifty to seventy-five percent sucrose, molasses is rich in calcium, iron, and potassium.

*Rice syrup* is a naturally processed sweetener made from sprouted brown rice. It is thick and mild-flavored.

*Stevia* is available in powdered or liquid form and is 30 times sweeter than sugar, noncaloric, and naturally derived from the stevia plant. Stevia has no impact on blood sugar levels, yeast-type conditions such as candidiasis, or IBS. Stevia can be used in conjunction with rice syrup in baking to further sweeten the finished product. Look for this sweetener in the "dietary supplement" section of your health food store.

*Sucanat* is a trademark name for "sugarcane naturally." It is the evaporated granules of sugarcane juice and molasses. It is 90 percent sucrose and a refined product. Use sparingly.

## STRESS LESSEN
### Groovin' and Cookin'

Cooking at home can be a wonderful, enjoyable experience. Turning the practice of cooking into a meditation will help to keep the focus on what is truly important—nurturing, joy, sharing, and the vital life force of food. Creating an atmosphere of relaxed fun in the kitchen can lead to a better cooking experience as well. Use music to change the atmosphere of your kitchen into a lively, calm, cheerful, or inspiring setting, depending on the food you're preparing.

- *Italian food:* Operas by Giuseppe Verdi, Gioachino Rossini, Giacomo Puccini
- *Mexican food:* Mariachi, salsa, merengue, *The Buena Vista Social Club* from Cuba
- *Baking:* Sing-along songs like the theme song from *Sesame Street* or *Putumayo Kids: Sing Along with Putumayo*
- *BBQ:* Country music, blues, jazz
- *Stir-fry:* Rock 'n' roll
- *Appetizers:* Disco classics or '50s and '60s lounge music
- *Salads:* Classic rock or new age

# MENTAL DETOX
## Sweet Stories

Sugar, honey, sweetie, cupcake—am I talking about a loved one or a sugary treat? The emotional realm of sugar addiction can have a powerful effect on our food cravings. Loneliness, fear, anxiety, stress, depression, and sadness are all emotions that can cause us to reach for a box of cookies hidden under our desks or stashed in the cabinet. What are these emotions you're feeling? Where do they come from?

**Exercise:** Using a blank sheet of paper, begin writing about your earliest childhood memories that involved sweets. Did your coach buy ice cream for the team when you won a game? Did your grandparents soothe a scraped knee with a lollipop? Did you and your mom share a box of chocolates when family squabbles erupted? Think about the ways in which you have used sugar in your life to make yourself feel better. Did sugar help to keep your mind off of an unhappy home life or childhood experience? Understanding where your ideas about sugar came from and what *sugar* means to you will help you to find the sweet things in life that don't come in a wrapper.

CHAPTER 6

# The Caffeine Crutch

## Week 3: Breaking the Habit
## Nutritional Issue: Caffeine

Most of us don't just enjoy a good cup of coffee (or tea) when we get up in the morning: We *need* one just to get the day rolling. That's because coffee and tea—like many other beverages, including soft drinks—are laced with caffeine, a powerful central nervous stimulant that is, arguably, the number one drug of choice for most Americans.

Caffeine acts on our brains much the way adrenaline does: It gives our nervous systems a quick boost that increases alertness (among other things), and this is the jolt from java that we all turn to first thing in the morning. The lift we get from coffee makes us feel less drowsy, less fatigued, and more able to sustain intellectual effort.

Caffeine enters the bloodstream through the stomach and small intestine, and its effects can be felt within 15 minutes of ingestion. Though caffeine is not stored in our bodies, the effects of a dose can be felt for up to 6 hours. The effects that caffeine has on our bodies are profound. Along with making us feel more "sharp," caffeine also increases heart rate, respiration, basal metabolic rate, gastroenteric reflexes, and the production of stomach acid and urine. It also relaxes smooth muscles such as the bronchial muscle.

Like so many other substances in our diet, caffeine is metabolized by the liver, and it is eventually released from the body in urine. And when we have too much caffeine, our liver—and other parts of our bodies—becomes overtaxed.

We all know what too much caffeine feels like: We get jittery and nervous, and our palms may even sweat. But too much caffeine also causes dizziness, nausea, headache, muscle tension, sleep disturbances, and irregular heartbeats. Extremely high doses (750 milligrams, or 7 or more cups of coffee a day) can induce all of the above reactions, plus anxiety attacks, severe drowsiness, ringing in the ears, diarrhea, vomiting, difficulty breathing, and even convulsions. It is actually possible to suffer a fatal overdose of caffeine (though this would entail drinking at least 80 cups of coffee in one sitting).

Much like our obsession with sugar, our addiction to caffeine forces us to ride a roller coaster of highs and lows. We take a cup of coffee to get us out the door in the morning, but by midmorning, many of us are feeling low again. This is when we traditionally take our first coffee break of the day and load up on our stimulant of choice, which is usually caffeine or sugar—or both. By late afternoon, when caffeine is no longer coursing through our veins, we tank up again. Before long, we can't get through the day without one, two, or many cups of coffee. Soon we're addicted to this stuff—and by "addicted," I mean *addicted,* as caffeine works on the same parts of the brain as amphetamines, cocaine, and heroin.

Aside from stimulating our metabolic systems in ways that aren't always desirable (are you literally shaking while you read this?), an infusion of caffeine into our brains signals to the pituitary gland that some sort of emergency must be happening. So it triggers our adrenal glands to produce adrenaline, which is the "fight or flight" hormone. When we have adrenaline running through us, our hearts beat faster and our blood vessels divert blood from surface areas and send it to our muscles. Our blood pressure rises, our stomach function slows, and the liver works to release sugar into our bloodstreams so we'll have the energy needed to respond.

Caffeine also increases dopamine levels in our brains, much the way amphetamines do. Dopamine is the neurotransmitter that activates the pleasure centers in our brains. This is another reason that we've become so fond of the stuff.

At the same time, caffeine keeps us up and awake because it interferes with a key chemical in the body called adenosine, which works as a natural sleeping pill. It's ironic, isn't it, that we take a drink to keep us up because we aren't getting enough rest largely due to the fact that what we're drinking (caffeine) kills our ability to sleep.

But what goes up must come down, and once the adrenaline leaves your system, you will feel more fatigued and more depressed than before you had that cup of coffee. So coffee does bring us up—but it also causes us to crash again. There is anything but balance in this caffeinated cycle we're slaves to. And detox is all about restoring balance.

## A Brief History of Caffeine

Caffeine is a naturally occurring chemical that is found in the leaves, seeds, or fruits of more than 60 plant species found all over the world. Many indigenous cultures, dating back to the Stone Age, figured out that chewing these leaves or berries would give them a buzz, and so they began using caffeine for ritual and medicinal purposes. The discovery of wild coffee cherries dates back to the 800s and is rooted in an Ethiopian legend about a sheep herder who saw the effect chewing the berries had on his animals. Two hundred years later, the beans were exported to the Arabian Peninsula, where coffee cultivation began in earnest. The Turks were the first people to make coffee into a drink. They would often flavor the brew with clove, cinnamon, cardamom, or anise. (The name coffee is a derivative of either the name of a region in Ethiopia called Kaffa or the Arabic term *qahway*, which literally means "that which prevents sleep." Both are credited as sources of the English word *coffee*.)

Though coffeehouses had existed in Turkey during the 13th century, the first known European coffeehouse didn't open until the mid-17th century in England. By the 18th century there were more than

2,000 coffee shops in London alone. Now, in the 21st century, you can't walk down an American street without bumping into a Starbuck's or a Dunkin' Donuts, or some other purveyor of coffee and tea.

Today, coffee is a seriously big business, with revenues of nearly $20 billion annually. But caffeine is showing up in more than just our cups. It is a chief ingredient in many medications, including over-the-counter headache remedies (caffeine causes blood vessels to constrict, thereby reducing bloodflow and pain). It is also added in significant amounts to other beverages, including soft drinks, sports drinks, and a new breed of beverage known as energy drinks (Red Bull et al). Caffeine is now even being added to bottled water! A 12-ounce can of soda contains 35 milligrams of caffeine, about one-third of what one finds in a cup of strong fresh-brewed coffee, which contains more than 100 milligrams of caffeine. Most diet sodas contain 40 milligrams of caffeine. Why is this stimulant put into soft drinks? The companies who make them say it is because it makes them taste better, but this is ludicrous: Before caffeine is chemically processed, it has a very bitter taste. In the 1920s, soft drink makers built their advertising campaigns by touting the addition of caffeine for its stimulating effects (originally, Coca-Cola had cocaine in it, but that practice was outlawed). Once the government questioned this practice, they decided to switch to the tactic of saying they add this stimulant for flavor.

## How We Become Coffee/Caffeine Junkies

I began drinking coffee when I worked at a drive-thru espresso hut in college. I would wake up 5 days a week at 5:00 A.M. and have my first cup when I started setting up the shop. This little cup of coffee, with its 100 milligrams of caffeine, gave me a hit of energy and woke up my senses and prepared me to tackle the day. Over the course of an average day, I would replenish my energy every few hours with another latte, another soda, or another cup of tea. Because caffeine doesn't build up in the body, it is excreted from our systems within a few hours. Once this would happen and the effects of the caffeine had worn off, my body and brain would quickly run down. I literally felt like my batteries were leaking. So I would grab another cup. This is how my addiction to the stuff began, and I bet my story isn't that different from yours. But coffee might not be your caffeine-source of choice. Consider the story of one of my clients, who came to understand her caffeine addiction in a roundabout way:

My client Sara repeatedly talked about her addiction to chocolate in our sessions together. Most afternoons while working at her desk, Sara would get cravings for sweet, dark chocolate that had to be satisfied by any means. Usually, she would find a piece of good-quality dark chocolate and continue on with her work. Trying to overcome this daily habit was causing Sara a lot of concern—why did she need this chocolate fix every day? We talked about her relationships, but she was happily dating at the time. Her career was heading in the right direction, and she was getting a good amount of creative outlet through her photography. As an experiment, Sara began picking up a cup of coffee in the afternoons during a short walk outside of her office—her reasoning was that she just needed some air, and the exercise would take her mind off the chocolate. Interestingly enough, as she began to drink coffee on a daily basis, her cravings for chocolate diminished, then disappeared. The caffeine in the chocolate was what Sara was really addicted to—it wasn't the creamy taste or texture. She was a caffeine addict.

In his book *Caffeine Blues,* Stephen Cherniske explains this in chemical terms: "Caffeine is, after all, a psychoactive drug, and human beings tend to crave substances that alter their state of mind—among them caffeine, morphine, nicotine, and cocaine. Indeed all of these alkaloids are chemically related and, while they produce widely different effects, all are poisonous."

Once we're on the caffeine roller coaster of high energy followed by a slump of low energy, we're locked into an endless addiction cycle. Your body begins to need and crave caffeine just to get itself back to a state of "normal." That's why I advocate for detoxing from caffeine, so your body can truly get back to a state of balance that isn't propped up by any kind of chemical dependency.

## BEYOND THE BRAIN: WHAT'S CAFFEINE DOING TO OUR BODIES?

We all know that caffeine offers us a mental boost, but what is it doing to the rest of the body? The overall consequences of regular coffee, soda, and tea consumption can be more harmful than must of us know. Until recently, modern medicine had not made the link between our morning cup and our deteriorating health. Evidence from recent studies has linked caffeine use with insulin resistance, adrenal exhaustion, liver and kidney problems, thyroid issues, and a sugar-craving cycle that seems unbreakable. Even casual consumption of caffeinated beverages has been shown to increase the risk of heart disease. Women especially should watch their caffeine habits, as caffeine causes valuable calcium to be lost through the urine. In addition, colas have a high phosphorus content, which also binds with calcium. Again, the calcium is leached out of the body through the urine, leading to increased risk of fractures and osteoporosis.

I have worked with several clients who report problems with insomnia and other sleep disorders. Why can't they sleep? One young woman, Barbara, talked about her erratic wake-sleep cycle—she worked the night shift and began to rely on a popular energy drink to wake her up and get her through work. By the time she returned home from work, she had consumed at least three Red Bull drinks— and now she couldn't sleep. Her productivity at work was affected, and her short-term memory was sketchy at best. Her mood was negative, and she began to feel depressed. Barbara turned to sugary treats to try to make herself feel better, adding to the already strong imbalance her body was dealing with. Instead of addressing the caffeine problem that was making her feel bad in the first place, she simply buried it under a sugar addiction. Now she felt worse than ever.

Insulin sensitivity has been linked with regular consumption of caffeine as well. When added to the already serious issues of hypoglycemia and diabetes, an increase in sensitivity to and imbalance of insulin is a major concern. The hormone epinephrine is also boosted by this drug in our cups. In addition to these already sobering facts, be aware that coffee is one of the most heavily sprayed crops for pesticides, and beans that are imported can be coated with unregulated pesticides used in foreign countries. These toxins, as well as dioxin and chlorine, which can leach out of white, bleached coffee filters, can add more than just a jolt to your morning cup of java.

Caffeine consumption, the little "monkey on our back," may also lead to a loss of aortic and vascular elasticity, which raises blood pressure. Caffeine causes our blood vessels to function in a very tense way, and large amounts of caffeine can lead to anxiety disorders, arthritis, and even vascular illnesses such as stroke. Coffee consumption has also been associated with raised estrogen levels, which some experts believe may lead to an increased risk for breast and endometrial cancer.

## IS CAFFEINE THE CULPRIT?

Our entire culture is, quite literally, sleepwalking through life. We're a nation of seriously sleep-deprived citizens, and researchers are just beginning to understand how crucial adequate sleep is to overall good health. In late 2004, researchers even began to make connections between insufficient amounts of sleep and obesity! Since 90 percent of us take in caffeine on a regular basis, couldn't there be a link between our caffeine consumption and our lack of sleep and, by extension, our problem with obesity?

The National Sleep Foundation (NSF) acknowledges that many of us reasonably rely on caffeine to help us overcome daytime sleepiness. But too much of it can seriously impact our ability to get an adequate night of rest. In the estimation of the NSF, anything beyond 250 milligrams a day (which is roughly a cup of coffee and two sodas) may start to affect sleep. Drinking or eating caffeine-rich foods and beverages right before bedtime, or taking medications that are high in caffeine, can increase the amount of time it takes to fall asleep and cause tossing and turning, can cause us to awake during the night, or can decrease total sleep time. Most adults need a minimum of 8 hours of sleep a night to maintain optimal health. But few of us are getting it. Cutting caffeine is a great way to get our sleep schedules back on track.

## CREATE A SANCTUARY FOR SLEEP

Creating a peaceful environment in which to sleep will entice you to make getting a good night's rest a priority. So, too, will engaging in healthy sleep habits before you hit the sack. Here are some tips.

- Don't eat foods or drink beverages laced with caffeine before bedtime, as caffeine will stay in your system for up to 6 hours and will disrupt your night's sleep.

- Exercise regularly, but not within an hour or two of bedtime.

- Go to bed at the same time every night and wake up at the same time every day. Your circadian clock thrives on this kind of routine.

- Don't eat for at least 1 to 2 hours before going to sleep. Also, focusing on a simple, light meal at the end of the day can ease digestion. Foods such as bananas, dates, figs, nut butters, or yogurt can be calming since they all contain tryptophan, which promotes sleep.

- Use your bedroom for sleep and sex only. Make it a distraction-free zone.

- Remove the television, the computer, and any other stress-inducing and distracting appliances from your bedroom.

- Hang heavy curtains to block out all light.

- Use earplugs to block out street noise or your partner's snoring.

- Take a warm bath before bed. It will ease your muscles and your mind.

- If you'd like a ritual snack before bed, have a cup of chamomile tea (if you are not allergic to ragweed) or catnip tea, as both have mildly sedating properties.

## KIDS AND CAFFEINE

I have lived in New York City for more than 5 years, and every year I see more fast-food-style coffee shops opening all the time, especially around universities, high schools, and hospitals. There are twice as many Starbucks on the island of Manhattan as there are McDonald's—and there are more McDonald's in New York City per capita than anywhere else in the country! It's virtually impossible for most New Yorkers to walk more than a block without being hit in the face with the smell of fresh brewed coffee.

Another sight that may be particular to New York is seeing teenagers and kids walking along drinking caffeine-loaded energy drinks, like Red Bull. These sleekly designed products are created with more caffeine than two cans of soda or more than six bottles of iced tea! Nutrition labeling laws require that if caffeine is added to a product, it must be listed on the ingredient list. However, there is no law requiring the listing of how much caffeine (the number of milligrams) is actually in the product.

According to the National Soft Drink Association, at least 60 percent of all middle and high schools sell soft drinks to students. Every year, more schools are making deals with these companies. Since 2000, more than 240 school districts have signed contracts with soda manufacturers to give them exclusive rights to sell kids their daily fix of caffeine. School administrators on the defensive ask what is wrong with selling sodas to kids—if it were dangerous, would the government allow these deals? Kids consume more food and beverages per body weight than adults do, and there simply isn't any research that shows, definitively, what kind of effect caffeine has on a child's body.

But with all the caffeine American kids are consuming, it's a wonder they can concentrate in class at all. The growing number of teens and even preteens who are taking prescription drugs for attention deficit disorder (ADD) and attention-deficit/hyperactivity disorder (ADHD) has skyrocketed in the last 5 years. More than four million U.S. teens are taking Ritalin or Adderall to help them focus and study. Strangely, this epidemic of attention problems hasn't afflicted most other countries. Could ADD be some kind of super-smart disease that doesn't cross borders? Or are our kids being drugged by too much caffeine and sugar in their foods?

## How to Get Off the "Caffeine Express"

With all of this new knowledge in hand about what caffeine is and what it does to your body, you're probably thinking it would be a good idea to get off the "caffeine express" as soon as possible. And you would be right—except that detoxing from caffeine should be done with care. There is no doubt that a caffeine-free life is a better life for your health, but caffeine is a very tough habit to break. For most of us, the withdrawal symptoms that hit us as soon as we deprive ourselves of coffee make the idea of kicking it for good too daunting to contemplate. I remember Morgan going through a few days of serious withdrawal after he quit his McDonald's diet, and it was very hard to watch. If you choose to quit caffeine cold turkey, be forewarned: It may hurt. Literally. Caffeine constricts the blood vessels in the brain, and once you remove the caffeine, the veins flex open and the blood pours forth, causing a terrible (albeit harmless) headache. You may also experience body aches, stomach problems, irritability, depression, and fatigue. Be gentle with yourself—you have been using a powerful drug for a long time, and once you're no longer ingesting it, your body will react immediately and forcefully to its absence.

The best way to detox from caffeine is to do it slowly, by gradually decreasing your intake of the drug. Don't beat yourself up for not being able to quit in 1 day—if quitting caffeine were that easy, we would all be free of it!

Here are some proven techniques for getting caffeine out of your life. Remember, go easy on yourself, and set realistic goals for reducing your consumption over time. Start by going "half and half" with a half-decaf, half-regular cup of coffee. Drink your usual number of these half-mixes daily for the first 4 days. In addition, drink a cup of regular water, hot or cold, for every cup of coffee you drink. This will keep your body properly hydrated, as dehydration is a common source of fatigue. On day 5, reduce the mixture to three-quarters decaf, one-quarter regular coffee. Continue this for another 4 days, continuing to drink a glass of water after each cup. Then you can make the switch to a full cup of decaf coffee, caffeine-free herbal tea, or other beverage. I recommend using "Swiss water process" decaffeinated coffee, which is processed with a nonchemical method of removing caffeine from the beans. Other decaffeination methods use chemicals in the process, and these chemicals are more likely to end up in your cup. The term "naturally decaffeinated" used on some brands of coffee is unregulated, so contact the manufacturer if you are unsure of whether or not they use chemicals in the decaffeination process.

For addicted tea drinkers, start weaning yourself by steeping your tea bag for less time. Alternate having a cup of regular tea with a cup of herbal or green tea, and you'll enjoy the same warm ritual without the caffeine. Continue working down your amount of black tea by replacing more and more cups with caffeine-free herbal tea or green tea. While green tea has one-third of the caffeine present in coffee, it also has a less bitter taste and has other beneficial effects on the body, so using it as a "transitional" drink while weaning yourself off of caffeine-rich black tea is a great option. Continue to hydrate with the following foods and liquids: good old-fashioned water, diluted fresh fruit and vegetable juices, herbal teas, soups, and whole fresh fruits and vegetables. Be aware that fruit juice has a high concentration of sugar, and sometimes people fall back on it as a crutch to get them through the caffeine blues.

Our culture has taught us to prefer and idolize beauty without effort, success without demands, and happiness without pain. In traditional Asian medical systems, light is always accompanied by the dark. It is the yin and yang of living. As winter proceeds into spring, our wholeness becomes defined by these contradictions of past and future, sour and sweet. Symptoms of withdrawal are a sign that the detoxification process is working—your body is releasing an artificial way of functioning and readjusting to its organic systems and state. If you think it would be helpful, allow yourself to retreat and care for yourself gently and kindly during this process. If you've been running yourself ragged on the treadmill of modern life, and you've used caffeine as the fuel to keep you going, it only makes sense that you may have to give yourself some space and time for detoxification to occur.

## TIPS FOR NATURALLY ENERGIZING YOUR BODY

In addition to slowly reducing and eliminating caffeine, what can you do to perk yourself up, get yourself motivated, and feel energetic? Here are a few tips on how to get moving.

- Hydrate, hydrate, hydrate. Drink plenty of water—get at least eight glasses a day.
- Walk it off. Feeling droopy at work? Take 10 minutes out of your lunch break to walk briskly around your building, to walk to your car and back, or to do a quick errand. Pumping your blood with oxygen, waking up your brain, and swinging your limbs will help awaken your body in a healthy way.
- Lower and then eliminate your intake of refined sugar. By detoxifying your body of sugar and caffeine at the same time, you stand a better chance of getting into your body's natural rhythms and keeping your energy steady.
- Stretch it out. Take 2 minutes at your desk to stretch your muscles. Raising your arms, touching your toes, arching your back,

## Herbs for Energy!

- Ginkgo biloba: Improves brain function by increasing circulation
- Gotu kola: Decreases fatigue and/or depression, stimulates central nervous system
- Lavender: Relieves stress and good for relieving headaches
- Licorice root: Supports adrenal gland function and mitigates endocrine exhaustion
- Maca: Increases energy and supports the immune system

or twisting your trunk can give you a quick shot of energy to get you through the afternoon.

- Deal with your stress. By facing and eliminating the areas of your life that are a source of stress, you will automatically feel lighter, more energetic, and less fatigued. Look at your whole life and address those areas that are holding you back from being your amazing, ultimate self.

## STRESS LESSEN
### Teatime Rituals

Legend has it that tea was invented by a Chinese emperor more than 5,000 years ago when some tea leaves accidentally blew into his pot of hot water. The tradition of serving tea to guests is an ancient ritual of welcoming, sharing, relaxation, and sustenance. The British have taken the ritual of teatime to another level by creating a complete daily meal around it. Teatime usually comes in the afternoon when life is transitioning from the workplace back into the home. Although business meetings, all sorts of celebrations, and simply visiting with friends are usual reasons for a "high tea," creating your own ritual with tea is a great way to carve out some quiet time during the day and take a break for some self-nurturing. A ritual created around tea drinking can be especially helpful for people who are trying to end their caffeine addiction since it fills the gap of a coffee break.

Perhaps creating a ritual of a *tea break* can help revive a tired office worker during the usual 3 o'clock energy lag.

- Create a special place for all your tea items. A secondhand tray or breakfast-in-bed tray will do nicely.

- Gather a small collection of tea items that are appealing to the eye as well as calming for your environment, including a small teapot, two or three teacups or mugs, teaspoons, and various herbal teas for different moods.

- Choose a 15- to 30-minute break during the day to sit down with your tea tray, hot water, and either a friend for conversation, a journal for reflection, or a good book.

- For a calming effect, try chamomile, Celestial Seasoning's Sleepy Time Tea, or Yogi Tea's Calming Tea.

# MENTAL DETOX
## Stress Test

Modern human beings are stressed to the max. Mental and physical pressures from career, relationships, commuting, and "dis-ease" combine to create incredibly powerful symptoms of overload. Explosive anger, sleeplessness, anxiety, depression, helplessness, and weight gain or loss are all outer signals that our minds are under too much stress. Read your body for these signs—is your daily stress causing your life to be extremely difficult and joyless?

Pinpointing and understanding the areas of your life that are causing you *distress* is a major step toward eliminating the pressure and learning to relax and enjoy life. Examination of your whole life will help you to do what you were designed to do: be a healthy, vibrant human being.

**Exercise:** Using a blank sheet of paper or journal, begin writing about all of the causes of stress in your life. Detail the physical and mental reactions that you have when faced with certain situations or people. Admitting the reasons for your irritation, whether they include an unfulfilling career, unhappy relationship, or not enough time for yourself, will help you to understand the emotional reasons for your stress-filled reactions. Learning to write about these issues can lead to better verbal communication with others about why you are upset. All of these factors line up to produce a straighter path toward solving problems, relaxation, and a de-stressed life.

# CHAPTER 7

# The Skinny on Fat

## Week 4: The Right Fat Does a Body Good
## Nutritional Issue: Dietary Fat

Here's a question: Do we need fat in our diets? Most of us equate fat that comes in foods with just one thing—being fat. But dietary fat is actually a necessary nutrient for the human body. Fat plays a role in blood clotting; absorption of vitamins A, D, E, and K; facilitating brain function; cell and hormone production; protecting vital organs; and providing energy. Fat is actually healthy—when we eat it in the right form and in the right measure. While the human body needs fats and fatty acids to function and thrive, our bodies don't produce them, so we must ingest them through our diets. The fact that we can't live without them has prompted the experts to label them as being *essential* to our health.

Fats, or *lipids,* are a class of substances that are not soluble in water. Greasy and slippery, fat provides a protective coating and lubrication for our organs and bones, and it is a form of transportation for all the myriad chemicals that make up our bodies. Also, just a little healthy fat goes a long way in balancing—and curbing—our appetites. Craving fat is natural—more than 50 percent of the calories in breast milk are from fat, which is crucial to a baby's brain and physical development. Most nutritional experts hold mother's milk up as an example of a "perfect food." It is important to remind ourselves that nature's most balanced and life-promoting food—breast milk—is made up mostly of fat.

Another reason why it's so important to include fats in our diets is that fats make food taste good! Clients often ask me why they are so attracted to the smell of cooking fat. Greasy, fried foods make our mouths water because we know that rich, satisfying food is near. It works as a taste enhancer, moving flavors around our tongues, fulfilling our desires for rich, full tastes. Some people who eat "nonfat" and "low-fat" diets have found that their appetites become insatiable—they can't get enough food, and so they binge on more and more low-fat and nonfat processed foods that have been heavily marketed to them by playing on their fears about fat. These low-fat and nonfat foods are manufactured with added sugar, salt, and additives to make up for the fact that they are lacking in natural taste.

Labels can be deceiving—and "low fat" can be an outright lie. When a product says "low fat," it is actually referring to the total calorie amount of fat per serving. Every gram of fat contains 9 calories. If a product claims to have only 1 gram of fat, that may sound like a very low amount. But what if the total calorie count per serving is only 18 calories? This means that the amount of fat per serving is 50 percent. And this is rarely a good thing. Most of us don't know to divide the total number of calories by the number of fat calories in a given food to figure out just how much fat that food contains. To help you work your way through the "low-fat" labeling maze, see the list of common food label terms in "FDA Rules for Fat on Food Labels" on page 99.

How do we tell the difference between a "good fat" and a "bad fat"?

Trying to make sense of fats is nearly impossible, given the confusing and often contradictory diet advice we've been given over the past 30 years. Like sheep, we follow one fad diet after another that either vilifies or elevates one nutrient over another, with the result

| FDA Rules for Fat on Food Labels |

## FDA Rules for Fat on Food Labels

- "Low Calorie": no more than 40 calories per serving
- "Reduced Calorie": 25 percent fewer calories than the regular product
- "Calorie Free": fewer than 5 calories per serving
- "Fat Free": no more than 0.5 gram of fat per serving
- "Low Fat": 3 grams of fat or fewer per serving
- "Free," "No," or "Zero": no amount or a trace amount of fat

being that we're constantly being pulled from one extreme to another, and always further away from a wholesome, well-balanced way of eating. We're told to follow a nonfat, then a low-fat, then a high-protein diet . . . then wait! make that a high-fat diet! It's no wonder that it's difficult to understand where fat fits into a healthy diet. Because of the way food is marketed to us, and how various fad diets seem to become gospel, we're constantly asking the wrong question about fat, which is: Is it good for us or bad for us? The question we should be asking is What kinds of fat are healthy and which are harmful?

## WHAT, EXACTLY, IS FAT?

While all fats have the same number of calories per gram (9), the chemical composition of fats can vary greatly. And this difference in chemical makeup has a profound effect on how the body metabolizes fats. The two main types of fat are saturated and unsaturated fats. Naturally, saturated fats are fat molecules that are saturated with hydrogen molecules. These fats are solid at room temperature. Fats that are missing molecules of hydrogen are known as unsaturated fats, and these are liquid at room temperature.

The mass-market food industry, however, has changed the very nature of saturated fats and made them even more harmful to us. In order to include fats in highly processed foods, it became necessary to figure out a way to turn liquid unsaturated fats into solid saturated fats. The way to do this was to artificially add hydrogen to these fats in a process known as hydrogenation. Why did the food industry need to come up with this trick? It would be impractical to try to package and sell cookies made with liquid fats—they would ooze and leak out of their packaging, and so their shelf life would be short. So the food industry decided the way to tackle the issues of longevity, shape, and ease of transport was to come up with a method for turning good, liquid fat into bad, solid fat and add it to most processed foods.

Hydrogenation doesn't just turn an unsaturated fat into a saturated fat; it also changes its molecular shape. When this happens, we're left with trans fat, which are, to most experts, the most harmful fats of all. These fats are difficult for our bodies to process and are commonly labeled as partially hydrogenated or just hydrogenated oils.

Nowadays, most fast-food restaurants use hydrogenated oils for deep frying and cooking, simply because they become rancid less quickly than unsaturated oils. Mass-produced baked goods such as doughnuts, cookies, and crackers also have high levels of trans fatty acids, unless their labeling tells us otherwise.

What's the problem with trans fat? The first clue as to why trans fats are dangerous is that they are not naturally occurring in food. Whatever type of fat we ingest becomes the type of fat we store in our bodies, so eating these "unnatural" fats causes our bodies to create a stockpile of toxic fat residue. Research shows that trans fat contribute to more cardiovascular problems than saturated fats. Trans fatty acids are artery clogging, increase blood levels of LDL, or "bad" cholesterol, and lower levels of HDL, or "good" cholesterol. Trans fat has also been linked to diabetes, heart disease, and hardening of the arteries and veins.

As I was writing this, in early 2005, it was announced that McDonald's Corporation settled a lawsuit brought by a group called BanTransFats.com. The restaurant chain has to pay $8.5 million, with $7 million going directly to the American Heart Association. That $7 million will be used specifically to help educate the public about the dangers of consuming foods high in trans fat, to encourage the food industry to use substitutes for partially hydrogenated oils, and to fund other activities that address the impact of trans fat on public health.

# FAT, TOXINS, AND YOUR LIVER

"Your liver has turned into pâté," Morgan's doctor announced, about 20 days into his 30-day fast-food diet. These are words you never want to hear from your medical advisor, and we were worried. Morgan's poor liver was being polluted with fat and toxins at an alarming rate—and this is a side effect most people never equate with eating this type of food. Even Morgan's doctors were shocked by this horrible development! Morgan was in danger of permanently ruining his liver. Dr. Isaacs urged him to stop the experiment immediately. To my horror, Morgan pressed on. How could this happen so quickly? How could Morgan's liver go from healthy to so sick in such a short amount of time? At first it didn't make sense, but just reviewing the processes your liver is involved in makes this all frighteningly clear. The liver is responsible for filtering the blood and extracting all the fat-soluble toxins that the kidneys can't handle. Morgan's food was overloaded with these toxins in the form of trans fat from all of the processed and fried foods he was buying from the drive-thru. His liver wasn't able to deal with this huge amount of toxic fat, so it was doing the only thing it could possibly do: It was storing this fat within its own tissue, causing it to be sick and bloated.

Normally, the gallbladder stores and releases bile, which is made by the liver and used for digesting fatty foods. However, the liver often has to reuse bile—even bile that has become tainted with the toxins from fatty foods. This bile, already rendered less effective because it is diluted with toxins, becomes less and less able to process the ongoing influx of toxins that a fast-food diet dumps on the liver. Meanwhile, the liver has to keep filtering blood, yet it has accumulated more toxins that have to be eliminated. The liver has to continue adding more toxins to the bile that it must reuse. When the bile recycles again, the liver is forced to squeeze in even more toxins. Eventually, both the bile and the liver are simply glutted with toxins, and their functioning begins to falter. This is what happened to Morgan. The more trans fat he ate, the more stressed his liver became (and the more taxed his gallbladder was), and the less able his body was to eliminate these fatty poisons.

Fortunately, removing these fat-associated toxins from our

bodies isn't as hard as you might think. Healthy oils and fats are actually (and ironically) great cleansers. Fats break down fats—so when you include healthy fats in your diet, you are ensuring that your body has the tools it needs to break down and eliminate stored fat-soluble toxins. The best way to get the healing benefits of healthy fats into your body is to cook for yourself at home. By preparing your own meals and ending the constant drive-thru and prepackaged food habit, you can easily eliminate these harmful trans and hydrogenated fats from your diet.

Instead of stocking your home cupboards with processed snack foods like chips, cookies, and crackers, transition to healthier and delicious convenience foods like the ones I recommend below.

- Air-popped popcorn drizzled with olive oil and sea salt
- Rice cakes with nut butters, apple butter, hummus, or tofu spread
- Homemade muffins and biscuits
- Tortilla chips made with non-hydrogenated oil
- Olives
- Trail mix: Create a mixture of nuts, seeds, and dried fruit.
- Edamame: Whole soybean pods are available in freezer packages. Boil for a few minutes (less than 10) and sprinkle with ½ teaspoon salt. This is a tasty, high-protein snack full of healthful fats.

Minimizing your intake of trans fat and hydrogenated oils will jump-start your detox and get your body back on track to functioning optimally. Once your liver is freed up from processing and eliminating trans fat, it can get to the work of detoxifying the other fat-soluble toxins that may be lurking around the fatty tissue in your organs and bloodstream. Learning where these "bad" fats are hiding on your plate is the next step to avoiding them. For Morgan it was easy—he stopped eating fast food and ate only the whole food meals we prepared at home. Once you've eliminated fast food from your diet, move on to clearing other highly processed foods from your pantry. Make an effort to avoid eating processed, packaged foods, and make it a priority to eat freshly prepared, homemade foods. When you make your own food, you have control over the quality of the ingredients, you get to cook your meal exactly how you want it cooked, and you give yourself a gift of nourishment and attention.

## Liver-Supportive Foods

If you sense at all that your liver is overtaxed, give it a boost by adding some or all of these foods to your diet.

- Alfalfa sprouts
- Burdock root
- Dandelion root and greens
- Fresh fruit and vegetable juices
- Green leafy vegetables
- Kidney beans
- Nuts and seeds, especially raw almonds
- Peas
- Raw salads
- Soybeans
- Spirulina
- Stir-fries cooked in a little good-quality olive oil

Following is a list of foods that hide fats well; try to avoid them whenever possible.

- Aerosolized whipped cream
- Canned franks and beans
- Coffee shop pastries: mostly mass-produced, these contain untold numbers of additives and trans fat
- Creamy dressings
- Fried foods: battered and fried vegetables; French fries (which are about 40 percent trans fatty acids); fried chicken, fish, and meats; and mozzarella sticks
- Gravies
- Hot dogs
- Hydrogenated and partially hydrogenated oil products: margarine and solid vegetable shortening and overprocessed vegetable oils (check label)

- Ice cream
- Imitation dairy products
- Mayonnaise
- Microwave popcorn
- Muffin and cake mixes
- Packaged potato and rice mixtures
- Peanut butter: read the label; look instead for unsweetened, nonhydrogenated nut butters (to make your own, see page 243)
- Processed meats: deli meats like bacon, bologna, and smoked and canned meats
- Processed snack foods: cakes, cookies, crackers, doughnuts, pastries, potato and corn chips (which can have as much as 30 to 50 percent trans fatty acids)
- Sausages
- Toaster pastries

While the foods listed above might seem obvious, other seemingly healthy foods like cereals can also contain trans fat. In order to avoid these toxins, you must become a food detective. Start reading your food labels and look for buzz words like *shortening, hydrogenated oil,* or *partially hydrogenated oil.* Remember, ingredients are listed on food labels in the order of highest content to lowest content. While some food companies are beginning to list the amount of trans fat in their products, many still do not, so you will benefit from doing a few seconds of math. By adding up the amount of fat in your box of cereal, doughnuts, or crackers (the individual listings of saturated, monounsaturated, and polyunsaturated fat), you can compare the total amount of fat per serving with the total fat listed on the label. When they don't match up, it is probably because of hidden trans fatty acids. Here's an example: 1 gram of saturated fat, 2 grams of monounsaturated fat, and 2 grams of polyunsaturated fat is 5 grams of fat. Compare that with the 10 grams of total fat listed, and the product is hiding 5 grams of fat somewhere. It is likely to be trans fat, since manufacturers have not yet been mandated by law to label them separately. Beginning in

January 2006, manufacturers will be required to list trans fat on their labels.

## WHAT ARE GOOD SOURCES OF HEALTHY FATS?

Knowing that fat is necessary for a healthy body and mind is great—so what is the best way to get healthy fats into your diet? Start with EFAs, or *essential fatty acids*. "Essential" means your body can't produce these special fats on its own, and so you must get them through food. Necessary for proper cell function, brain development, a healthy nervous system, and hormone production, EFAs are crucial to detoxification as they transport fat-soluble vitamins around the body. A diet like Morgan's, which was full of saturated fats and processed vegetable oils, creates huge obstacles for the body in processing the EFAs which are so very important.

EFAs are found naturally in plant sources such as unrefined flax oil, pumpkinseed oil, nuts like walnuts, and vegetables such as green purslane. They are also found in fish that feed on EFA-rich seaweeds. Herring, mackerel, salmon, sardines, and sprat are especially good fish sources of EFAs. Increased EFA consumption has been found to lessen water retention and to reduce the risk of kidney problems, celiac disease, cystic fibrosis, inflammatory bowel disease, cardiovascular disease, strokes, and cancer. These oils are very delicate and should not be heated or cooked. You can add them to your diet by using these oils to make delicious salad dressings, dips, or light sauces. EFAs are incredibly helpful when detoxing, but they have a limited shelf life and are damaged and destroyed by exposure to heat and light. Purchase EFA-rich oils in small amounts, and buy only those that are bottled in dark, black, or opaque containers. Don't store them near heat sources, such as near the oven or on top of the refrigerator.

Whole nuts and seeds are nature's powerhouses of energy, protein, minerals, and natural fats. Keeping a container of homemade trail mix at your desk or in your kitchen can be a great alternative to a candy or cookie jar. Nuts are great sources of EFAs and vitamin E, both of which protect the nerves and nervous system. If you have trouble digesting nuts but would like to eat them, try soaking them overnight to activate the sprouting process. In the morning, strain and dry them and either roast them or eat them raw. Chewing nuts well will also ease their digestion. High in calories, nuts and seeds should be eaten in small amounts, but no healthy diet should exclude them.

Chia seeds and flaxseeds are the richest sources of EFAs. These seeds should be lightly ground using a coffee grinder, blender, or mortar and pestle to access all of the EFAs without damaging them.

Proper storage and use of nuts and seeds is important. Because of their high fat content, the oils can become rancid. Hollow-centered nuts should be discarded, as well as any nuts or seeds with mold, black spots, or a rancid smell. Storing nuts and seeds in a cool, dark place, or in the refrigerator or freezer, will slow oxidation of their oils. Buying nuts and seeds with their shells intact is a good way to protect them longer from light's harmful effects, and when they're still in the shell and kept in a cool, dark place, they will keep for about a year.

Cooking with high-quality fats and oils is the best way to ensure that what you eat will not harm your body and that it will actually promote detoxification. Find and cook recipes that use preparation methods like broiling, grilling, poaching, roasting, steaming, and stir-frying. These methods tend to use less fat and less heat. Recipes and ingredient lists that use terms like *breaded, buttered, cream, fried,* and *gravy* most often have a higher fat content and use fats in harmful ways.

Oils are manufactured and extracted in different ways, and some ways are definitely less toxic than others to our bodies. Here's a quick primer on the various techniques used to extract or process oils, beginning with the more healthful techniques.

**EXPELLER OR PURE PRESSED.** Expeller pressing is a chemical-free mechanical process that extracts oil from seeds and nuts. This method is far less toxic than the hexane-extraction method that is widely used in the food oil industry. (Hexane is a highly flammable gasoline-like solvent that nuts are drenched in in order to extract the oils from the seeds. The hexane is then "evaporated" off the nuts in a high-heating process. Hexane is categorized by the Environmental Protection Agency as a "hazardous air pollutant.") Seeds containing oil, like olive pits, are crushed with a mechanical press. The oil is squeezed out without the use of high temperatures or chemicals. A bottle must be labeled cold pressed, expeller pressed, unrefined, natural, or crude to be considered such. Though no heat is applied to the nuts or seeds, the pressure from the expelling process does produce heat from friction, which can damage the oil and cause it to oxidize and break down eventually. All oils, however, are fragile and are also prone to deterioration, and so those harvested by expeller or pure-pressed processes are still a good bet.

**ORGANIC.** These oils are made without the use of potentially hazardous chemicals, which can carry over into your food. The plants these organic oils are derived from have not been sprayed with pesticides, which can also end up as stored, fat-soluble toxins in your body. By spending a few extra dollars on organic oils, you can be assured that you are avoiding extra toxins and therefore extra stress on your body.

And, in the "not so good" category, we have:

**REFINED.** These oils are highly processed with chemical compounds to extend their shelf lives. Refining processes use bleaches, phosphoric acid, chemicals, and caustic sodas to create these oils— if the label does not list how the oil was extracted, it was most likely refined.

When you're shopping for oils, do read the label and look for key words like *unrefined* or *organic*. Also, chose an oil that is bottled in dark or opaque glass, as this will protect the oil from light and oxidation. Stay away from oils that are in clear bottles since inert gases are usually added to inhibit oxidation and the spoiling of the oil.

Finally, here are some quick tips for storing your cooking oils.

- Store unopened bottles in a cool, dark place.
- Refrigerate oils after opening, except olive oil.
- Never reuse oils that have been used for deep frying.
- Never use or consume an oil that smells rancid.
- Do not add new oil to a bottle of older oil.
- Do not heat oils to the smoking point.

## THE BEST COOKING FATS

Using proper oils that don't degrade while you cook is important when you're detoxing your menus. I have chosen to avoid using sev-

# Smoke Point Table for Oils

| OIL (UNREFINED) | TEMPERATURE | USE |
|---|---|---|
| Canola | Up to 120°F/49°C | Cold preparations: condiments/salad dressings |
| Flaxseed | Up to 120°F/49°C | Cold preparations: condiments/salad dressings |
| Walnut | Up to 120°F/49°C | Cold preparations: condiments/salad dressings |
| Pumpkin | Up to 212°F/100°C | Low heat: sauces/baking* |
| Safflower | Up to 212°F/100°C | Low heat: sauces/baking |
| Sunflower | Up to 212°F/100°C | Low heat: sauces/baking |
| Almond or Brazil nut | Up to 325°F/163°C | Medium heat: light sautéing |
| Hazelnut or pistachio | Up to 325°F/163°C | Medium heat: light sautéing |
| Olive, extra-virgin | Up to 325°F/163°C | Medium heat: light sautéing |
| Sesame | Up to 325°F/163°C | Medium heat: light sautéing |
| Coconut | Up to 375°F/190°C | High heat: baking/browning/frying |

*When baking to temperatures up to 325°F/163°C, the moisture keeps the inside temperature under 212°F/100°C.

Table from The Natural Gourmet Cookery School and Omega Nutrition, 1995 eral popular oils for other reasons as well. Peanut oil is not available in organic varieties, and some studies indicate that it may contribute to atherosclerosis in some animals and may contain aflatoxins, or toxic fungus contamination. Canola oil is also the subject of much debate. The refined version is good for high-temperature cooking, but it's refined with chemicals that should be avoided. The unrefined version of canola oil is suitable only for cold preparations like salad dressings; it shouldn't be heated because of its delicate essential fatty acids. It is also difficult to find an unrefined, organic version that is stable for long periods. Corn oil is also highly processed and tainted with pesticides. I choose to avoid these oils and use mainly extra-virgin olive oil, coconut oil, and sesame oil when I cook.

For years, tropical oils, such as coconut oil, have been vilified in the health media because of their high saturated fat content. I agree that processed, refined tropical oils are dangerous—just as processed and refined vegetable oils, such as hydrogenated margarine, are. However, unrefined organic coconut oil has some distinct and powerful health benefits that should be promoted. Unrefined coconut oil remains stable at higher temperatures, making it ideal for occasional baking and frying. This stability stops the oil from creating free radicals, the terrorist molecules that wreak havoc on our cells. Other vegetable oils that are lower in saturated fat break down at high temperatures and are better suited for quick-cooking methods such as sautéing and for salad dressings. Coconut oil is also lower in calories than most fats and oils, and it's a great source of lauric acid, which has been shown to enhance the immune system and is helpful for people with candida overgrowth. Strong anecdotal evidence about the benefits of coconut oil can be found in tropical traditional cultures all over the world. These cultures, including people from Thailand, the Philippines, Sri Lanka, Africa, India, and parts of South America, use unrefined coconut oils and yet they have lower levels of cholesterol, heart disease, and diabetes than people in the United States and other Western cultures have. Only after a modern, Western-style diet has been introduced to these cultures do incidences of these diseases increase.

The main source of fat in the heart-healthy, universally acclaimed diets of the Mediterranean region is extra-virgin olive oil, which is widely available here. Extra-virgin olive oil has a wonderful taste, a pleasant aroma, and great health benefits. High in vitamin E and monounsaturated fats, olive oil is the most stable vegetable oil after coconut oil. Used to support the liver, olive oil also lowers LDL cholesterol levels. "Extra virgin" refers to the fact that this oil is the first pressing of the olives, which is the best tasting. Olive oil does not need to be refrigerated, as this can cause it to solidify, but do store it in a cool dark place (not over the oven).

Sesame oil has a wonderful flavor and is used in traditional Asian and Indian cooking and is great for quick sautéing. High in both monounsaturated and polyunsatured fats, sesame oil contains a natural antioxidant, "sesamol," which stops the oil from turning rancid. Used to ease constipation, sesame oil is also wonderful for cracked skin due to dryness, and as a topical remedy.

Nut and seed oils like walnut, almond, and hemp are all gaining popularity for their distinct flavors, aromas, and lovely tastes. Because of their high fatty acid content they are delicate, so do not heat or cook with these oils. Use them on salads, on baked potatoes, and drizzled over food just before serving.

## Weighing In on Exercise

Ayurveda is an ancient school of medicine from India, dating back to around the 5th century B.C. Like Traditional Chinese Medicine, Ayurvedic medicine sees human health as a whole picture. Every person can be ascribed an individual body type that can be described as one of the three *doshas:* vata, pitta, and kapha. The *vata* body type is usually thin and small-boned, with visible joints and dry skin and hair. This person is more susceptible to the cold and nervousness—think Woody Allen. The *pitta* person is more athletic, muscular, fiery, and active, and he or she has a big appetite for living—think Morgan. The *kapha* person is usually heavyset and tends to be steady and slow-moving, but he or she is more grounded than the flighty vata person—think Winston Churchill. These are extremely simplified definitions, and several books have been written that can be helpful for determining your body type in this way. Many people are often a combination of two of the three doshas and can exhibit balanced and imbalanced symptoms.

Choosing an exercise that is right for your dosha can be helpful to bring balance to your body and mind.

*Vata exercises:* Grounding and strengthening with weight lifting and Pilates

*Pitta exercises:* Calming and relaxing physical exercises like yoga and Pilates

*Kapha exercises:* Get moving with cardiovascular exercises

To read more about self-testing and further explore the world of Ayurvedic medicine and body typing, see the books listed in "Additional Reading" on page 282.

## STRESS LESSEN
### Seventh-Inning Stretch

Simple stretching has an amazing impact on our stressed-out bodies and minds. Stretching our muscles keeps us limber and toned, and it also makes more formal exercising more effective and safe. Moving our muscles and bodies in different ways helps to *twist* and *squeeze* our tissues so that our circulation is improved. These movements also allow the body to remember its original shape and to settle into a more comfortable alignment. A good 5-minute stretch can calm the mind during a stressful day, as the body begins taking over the inner conversation happening inside the brain. "Mmmm, that side stretch feels good" begins to replace our worries over the latest spreadsheet or unreturned phone call.

- First sit quietly with your hands resting on your belly and close your eyes for 30 seconds. Breathe in deep, slow breaths, counting to four on the inhale, hold for two counts, and then exhale for four counts. This will allow you to center your focus and energy.

- Stand up and raise your arms above your head. Reach for the sky, first with one hand and then the other. Look up and feel your sides stretching as you reach. Reach 10 times with each hand.

- With your hands limp at your sides, slowly begin to bend forward at your waist and let your head hang forward. Allow your arms to hang down and breathe deeply seven times. Slowly stand back up with your knees slightly bent.

- Sit straight up in a comfortable chair and place your hands on your knees. Curl your back slowly and allow your head and neck to relax forward. Hold for three breaths, and slowly straighten up and push your chest slightly forward. Hold for three breaths and repeat seven times.

## MENTAL DETOX
### The Fat of the Land

Living up to the image of perfection that we see every day in the media is impossible: Even the Hollywood stars and runway models are pressured to constantly look better, younger, and slimmer. When the "beautiful people" don't even think that they look good enough, how are the rest of us supposed to feel? Imagine if no one had to think about how they looked or dressed anymore—if all of a sudden, no one judged themselves or you on your looks. Imagine harnessing all the energy that is wasted on feelings of inadequacy and fear of not being accepted and putting it to better use. This kind of shift in thinking could change the world.

Exercise: Using a blank page in a journal, write a love letter to your body. Tell it how soft, firm, long, grand, pretty, sexy, silky, strong, and wild it is. Marvel in the magic that happens just below your skin every second. Your heart never forgets to beat—thank it for keeping you alive. Your lungs never forget to breathe—thank them for always remembering to fill. Rejoice in the magic of the blood flowing through your veins, the miracle of cell division, and the divine good luck that gave you brown or blue eyes. Be in awe of the million small movements that happen inside of you every day that you don't even know are happening. Embrace the body that you have—it's the only one you'll ever get, so cherish it.

# A Carb Is Not a Carb Is Not a Carb

## Week 5: Getting a Handle on Carbohydrates
## Nutritional Issue: Carbohydrates

Carbohydrates are probably the nutritional staple that we get the most mixed messages about. For a time, we were encouraged to eat a diet loaded with carbohydrates. Now, the rage is to promote a high-protein/low-carbohydrate way of eating. But I would argue that when it comes to carbohydrates, talking about quantity is simply missing the point. Sure, you should be mindful of how many carbs you take in (living on bread and pasta isn't a healthy, nontoxic diet), but what you should really focus on is what type of carbs you're eating. Then you'll know whether you're eating carbs that will boost—or bust—your health.

Carbohydrates are necessary fuel if the human body is to function and thrive, and they are the main source of energy for our brains and muscles. While your diet may be full of refined carbohydrates, the unrefined, whole grain varieties are the real powerhouses of energy and lasting stamina. We metabolize whole grains in ways that are really beneficial to our bodies. Imagine that the way the body breaks down whole grains is like an IV drip: Because whole grains have high fiber content, these foods break down slowly, over time, so the sugar/energy in them is delivered to our bodies in a nice, steady, and healthful flow that can last hours. Compare that to how highly processed carbs are metabolized: They explode like a grenade inside, sending your blood sugar level sky-high only then to plummet like so much shrapnel, leaving you feeling lousy. Fast. Learning to love and eat the "whole grain" is an important step in moving away from one of the greatest dangers in the standard American diet and toward the detoxifying and fortifying benefits of a more wholesome diet. Whole grains can be extremely beneficial and have been used over centuries to help a lot of people detox and lead healthy lives.

Highly refined carbohydrates, including white flour, white sugar, and other simple sugars, are much different than the carbohydrates we consume when we eat whole grains, whole grain products, beans, and vegetables. How many people can say that they have been overeating brown rice and millet for 20 years and are now experiencing diabetes and obesity? According to the USDA, in the 1970s, Americans consumed 136 pounds of flour and refined cereal products per person per year. Today we're stuffing down 200 pounds per person per year. That's a 68 percent increase in refined carbohydrate consumption per person in just one short generation. It's true that at the molecular level all carbohydrates perform the same function in our bodies, whether we get them from candy bars or whole grain porridge. However, the carbs that come from whole grains contain fiber, which has been stripped from the husk of refined grains, and vitamins and minerals, which have been purged from the germ of refined grains, leaving only the starchy middle of the grain. The effect this has on the way the body processes this tampered-with carb is dramatic. Without the fiber to slow the breakdown of the molecules, and without the benefits of the innate essential vitamins and minerals, we're left with an empty carb that is metabolized immediately as straight sugar.

# What's the Difference between a Refined and an Unrefined Carbohydrate?

Do you remember making papier-mâché projects in arts and crafts class? The usual tools were strips of newspaper and a bowl of paste. That paste was made of a simple, cheap combination of ingredients: just standard white flour and water. It was sticky, it was gooey, and it worked like glue that hardened in no time. Now think about the last time you ate a piece of white bread or other refined-flour product. The flour in that white bread, once it was moistened with your saliva, became like that pasty glue, and this is what was sent into your digestive system: a gummy, nutrient-poor glob of starch. This is what your digestive system looked forward to processing. It's not tough to imagine how little nutrition was drawn from this ball of sticky matter, or how difficult it was for your body to finally eliminate it.

What's been "refined" out of these processed carbohydrates are all the beneficial nutrients that nature originally put into them. The bran, the fiber, and most of the vitamins and minerals have been stripped away, leaving a bland, white, longer-lasting and shelf-stable product. White flour has only 20 percent of the vitamins and minerals and 25 percent of the fiber of the original wheat kernel. That's why a lot of bread products are "enriched" with vitamins and minerals—they don't contain enough to mention otherwise. Whole wheat flour still contains the hull, germ, and bran of the grain and offers more fiber and nutrients. I look forward to the day when fast-food restaurants offer whole grain buns and fiber-rich side dishes to their customers, instead of the empty carbs that they now push on us so aggressively.

Now that we've talked a little bit about carbohydrates, why don't you take a minute to ask yourself if you might be eating too many of the refined, highly processed variety.

One way to distinguish between carbohydrates that harm us and carbohydrates that heal us is to think about their fiber content. Products that are made out of refined white flour and white sugar usually have very little fiber and are very processed. Fiber-filled carbohydrates are better for you than those with little or no fiber. Fiber

## TOO MUCH OF A BAD THING: ARE YOU EATING THE WRONG KIND OF CARBS?

- Do you feel bloated or tired after eating a meal with bread or pasta?
- If yes, are those feelings stronger if you eat a whole grain bread versus a refined, white flour product? (*Note:* Some people are very sensitive to whole grains and actually do feel bad after eating them.)
- Do you crave refined carbohydrates like white bread, white pasta, and white sugar?
- Do you get afternoon headaches after a lunch containing breads or pasta?
- When you eat white bread, white pasta, or white rice, do you feel hungry for more of the same?

If you answered "yes" to any of these questions, you need to re-think what kinds of carbs you're putting into that beautiful body of yours.

provides a barrier for your digestive system—otherwise the carbohydrates get turned into sugar immediately. Most Americans eat around 12 grams of fiber a day, while the recommended daily intake ranges from 20 to 45 grams. Yet we are overconsuming carbohydrates! Whenever you reach for a box of cereal, a loaf of bread, or any other product made with flour (pastas, etc.), always reach for the brand that lists whole wheat or another whole grain as the first ingredient. And also check the fiber content and go with the one that has the most fiber per serving.

In the last several years, a more sophisticated method has emerged to help us understand which carbs are good and which are bad. This is what is known as the glycemic index, or GI. The glycemic index rates how many readily available sugar is in a particular food. This, in turn, indicates how quickly that food will affect your blood sugar level. White bread, potatoes, and refined cereals, which are rapidly digested, create a surge in blood sugar levels, and so these are classified with high GI ratings. Foods with low GI ratings, such as vegetables, whole grain products, and beans are metabolized more slowly, largely because of their fiber content. These low-GI foods don't cause drastic changes in blood sugar levels and thereby eliminate the highs and lows that can lead to excess snacking and sugar cravings. Making a simple switch in the foods you eat can have a profound effect on your health. For example, eating brown rice instead of white rice will do wonders for controlling your blood sugar level. So will switching from white bread to whole grain bread. Plus, the extra fiber in these foods will expand in your stomach, so you will feel full faster and longer after eating whole grain products. When you're buying whole grain products, continue to be a good food detective and watch out for any ingredients that you are trying to avoid.

Fiber supplements can also be helpful in eliminating the toxic wastes that build up in our bodies when we eat a diet of highly refined carbs. But supplements aren't magic bullets: The best way to ensure that your body is getting the kinds of carbs it needs to run smoothly and stay "clean" is to keep eating whole grains, beans, vegetables, and fruits that give you the extra dose of fiber needed to clean out your system. The natural foods with the highest amounts of fiber are lentils; black, kidney, and lima beans; chickpeas; potatoes with the skin; peas; non-instant oatmeal; pears and apples with the skin; Brussels sprouts; and peaches.

## How to Read Labels on Carbohydrate-Rich Foods

- "Multigrain" means that a bread or cereal is made from more than one grain (like oats, rye, or wheat), but it doesn't mean the grains are *whole* grains. The grains could all be refined, making them as low in fiber and beneficial *phytochemicals,* the plant chemicals that contain protective, disease-preventing compounds, as the grains in white bread.

- Avoid instant rice and boxed, flavored rice mixes. They usually contain preservatives, sugar, and flavorings. You can make these dishes yourself at home at less cost and with more healthful and wholesome ingredients.

- "Made with whole grains" is another common label lie. The label is not required to list *how much* whole grain is in the food. The main ingredients could really be refined flours, with a bit of whole grain thrown in.

- Products labeled as "whole grain" must contain 51 percent whole grain by weight.

- Food served for immediate consumption, such as that served in hospital cafeterias and on airplanes, and ready-to-eat food that is not for immediate consumption but is prepared primarily on site—for example, bakery, deli, and candy store items, or items that are mass-produced and sold by food service vendors, mall cookie counters, sidewalk vendors, and vending machines—are all exempt from nutrition labeling. *Buyer beware.*

- Look at the "total carbohydrate" figure and the ingredient list to determine how healthy a bread product really is. "Dietary fiber" and "sugar" will be listed under "total carbohydrate." It's best to choose a bread with higher amounts of fiber and lower amounts of sugar. Read the ingredient list and avoid any breads with high levels of added sugar like high fructose corn syrup.

## COMMON GRAIN ALLERGIES: WHEAT, CORN, AND CELIAC DISEASE

Food allergies often go undiagnosed unless they're life-threatening, like the serious anaphylactic shock that occurs when one is allergic to peanuts or shellfish. Three of the most common food allergies are wheat, corn, and gluten, and these affect far more people than have been diagnosed. According to the International Food Information Council (IFIC), the top eight food allergies are wheat, milk, eggs, peanuts, tree nuts, fish, shellfish, and soy. (Though corn isn't on the IFIC's list of top food allergens, I encounter many people with a sensitivity to this grain. Corn, especially in the form of corn syrup, is a component in many highly processed foods, and we are reacting to it.) In addition to corn allergies, red meat, sugar, and tannin allergies also seem to affect many people.

Celiac disease, also known as celiac sprue, is genetic and affects the digestive system. People who have celiac disease cannot stomach gluten, which is a protein found in wheat, rye, spelt, triticale, Kamut, some oats, and barley. When people with celiac disease eat gluten, their immune systems react by damaging the *villi* in the small intestine. Nutrients from food move into the bloodstream through villi, so a person can become malnourished if he or she suffers from celiac disease.

For people with celiac disease, which is an autoimmune disorder, gluten is poison. The disease can be found in infants who fail to thrive, or it can be triggered later in life, brought on by severe stress, infection, surgery, pregnancy, or childbirth. Symptoms of celiac disease include frequent abdominal bloating and pain, diarrhea, weight loss, pale stool, anemia, gas, depression, fatigue, joint and bone pain, seizures, osteoporosis, painful skin rash, missed menstrual periods, muscle cramps, and tooth enamel damage.

Studies cited by the National Institutes of Health (NIH) show that celiac disease affects 1 in 133 Americans, though the NIH admits that the actual number is probably higher. The disease could be underdiagnosed in the United States because celiac symptoms are often attributed to other problems, many doctors are not knowledgeable about the disease, and only a few laboratories are experienced in testing for celiac. Celiac disease is sometimes misdiagnosed as another disease, such as irritable bowel syndrome (IBS), Crohn's disease, ulcerative colitis, diverticulosis, depression, chronic fatigue syndrome, or an intestinal infection. An antibody test or a biopsy performed by a doctor can detect celiac.

Living well with celiac disease involves following a gluten-free diet. Avoiding all foods that contain gluten will stop further damage and symptoms for most people and will heal their intestines. This diet is a lifetime deal, as celiac sufferers never recover from their "allergy" to gluten. A gluten-free diet isn't as hard to follow as it was in the past, and noticeable improvement is usually seen in about 2 weeks. New gluten-free products are appearing all the time, and breads, pastas, and cereals made from potato, rice, soy, and bean flours are available in a wide variety. Look out for hidden sources of gluten in food additives, preservatives, medicines, processed foods, and even mouthwash! Learning to eat "all over again" can be a challenge, but with practice, checking ingredient labels and asking chefs in restaurants if their dishes contain gluten will become second nature.

People who are allergic to wheat have negative responses only to wheat protein. These individuals can eat other gluten-containing grains, and many can tolerate Kamut or spelt, both ancient relatives of wheat that are used as a whole grain or flour. Experts estimate that there are as many as 3 million to 10 million wheat allergy sufferers in this country. I suggest that you monitor your own response to wheat to see if you might be undiagnosed with this food allergy.

Corn is everywhere—it is used as a filler, sweetener, and common side dish in most restaurants and homes. The overabundance of corn, in my opinion, is leading us to become sensitive and allergic to it, and corn is now one of the top 10 food allergens. The overuse of cornstarch, cornmeal, and high fructose corn syrup in most processed foods makes it difficult to avoid corn, so people with this allergy must be careful and prepare most of their own food. Reading labels closely will show you that even peanut butter, processed meats, imitation cheeses, and baby food can contain corn products. Dextrose—found in French fries, fish sticks, and potato puffs—dextrin, dextrate, maltodextrin, caramel, and malt syrup are also probable sources of corn. Caramel flavoring is often made with corn syrup, as is root beer and maple and nut flavors for ice creams, candy, and pastries. Even marshmallows contain corn—cornstarch is added to keep the sugar and baking powders from clumping. A terrific alternative to cornstarch is kudzu root, or kuzu, which is used in China and Japan just like we use cornstarch in America. Use ½ to ¾ teaspoon of powdered kudzu or ½ to 1 teaspoon of arrowroot per cup of liquid in recipes to replace cornstarch.

## WHAT'S SO GREAT ABOUT WHOLE GRAINS?

Whole grains are powerful sources of energy, so eating a wide variety of whole grains will maximize your exposure to the most diverse array of benefits. Whole grains are also great sources of fiber, minerals, protein, and vitamins. High in complex carbohydrates, with a rich amino-acid profile, whole grains keep their bran, fiber, germ, and endosperm. Whole grain carbohydrates also have fewer calories from fat. A study of health professionals at the Harvard School of Public Health showed that people who eat more whole grains weigh less than those who don't. The findings showed that 40 grams of whole grains a day cut weight gain in middle-age participants by as much as 3.5 pounds. Forty grams equals 1 cup of oatmeal, ¾ cup of brown rice, or three to five slices of whole grain bread. Similar studies show that eating whole grains cuts the risk of developing heart disease, diabetes, and obesity. Remember, one of the "diet" benefits of whole grain foods, as compared with refined-flour products, is that the bran, germ, and starchy endosperm still contained in the unrefined grain make us feel full faster.

All of us react differently to grains in our diets, and some people who are seriously addicted to refined carbohydrates may have strong reactions when they switch over to whole grain carbs. Grain sensitivities, besides celiac disease, can cause fatigue and bloating and can ignite cravings for more grains and carbohydrates. Eating smaller portions of grains once every few days is the best way to introduce them if your diet has been seriously devoid of them until now. Also, while whole grains are an excellent source of complex carbohydrates, some people cannot digest them well. By soaking grains overnight and then cooking them and preparing them with herbs and spices, grains become easier to digest and faster to prepare.

## Self-Test for Grain Sensitivities

To determine whether or not you are allergic to a particular grain, have a small portion of the grain for breakfast and do not add anything to it—no sweetener or milk, no fruit, and no nuts. Consume nothing else except water, not even a cup of tea or coffee. Take down notes about how you are feeling beginning about an hour later. Then take notes every hour for the next 2 hours. Do you feel bloated or tired? Foggy? Sleepy? Do you have a headache? Any of these symptoms can indicate sensitivity to the grain, and therefore it should be avoided. This self-test is a great way to get in touch with your body's reactions to certain foods.

If several grains cause you bad reactions, you should consider getting tested by a doctor for celiac disease and possible blood sugar imbalances. There are several tests that a doctor can administer to determine if you are allergic to certain foods. In a skin-prick test, a diluted extract of the suspected food is placed on the skin, which is scratched or punctured. A blood test can provide information similar to skin testing, although both forms of testing have been disputed by the National Institute of Allergy and Infectious Diseases. One of the best ways to avoid wheat-related intolerances is to use a *rotation diet,* where you restrict wheat-containing products to once every 4 days.

Whether gluten intolerant, allergic to certain grains, or simply

# Great Grains!

When we hear the word *grain,* most of us think wheat, corn, and maybe rye. But there is a whole world of grains available to us that are highly nutritious and delicious. Here's a list of my favorites.

**AMARANTH:** Higher in calcium and protein than cow's milk, amaranth was the staple grain of the Aztecs in South America. Highly nutritious, amaranth is also a good source of fiber, lysine, B vitamins, zinc, copper, and iron. Used medicinally to help congested lungs.

**BARLEY:** Used medicinally to support the gallbladder and digestive and nervous systems, barley also stimulates the liver and lymphatic system. High in fiber and great for bowel cleansing, barley helps prevent dietary cholesterol absorption. Barley miso, made with fermented soy paste, known as *mugi,* has been found to reduce tumors and body fat.

**BUCKWHEAT:** Not a true grain but really a grass seed in the same family as rhubarb, buckwheat is one of the most filling grains used for stabilizing blood sugar levels. Gluten-free, buckwheat neutralizes toxic acidic wastes in the blood. Good for circulation and used by the Japanese for its medicinal effect on the kidneys. Japanese soba noodles are made of buckwheat. High in calcium, protein, and vitamins B and E.

**CORN:** High in vitamins A, B, and C, calcium, folate, magnesium, phosphorus, potassium, and iron, corn also contains several phytochemicals. It is, however, one of the top 10 food allergens. People with corn allergies might do well with blue corn products and air-popped popcorn. Corn has been used medicinally for heart disease, blood sugar stabilization, and sexual weakness.

**KAMUT:** A relative of wheat, Kamut is tolerated by many people who are allergic to wheat. Use the whole grain for hearty dishes, or use the flour for homemade baked goods.

sensitive to insulin fluctuations, some people will do better by focusing on nongrain sources of complex carbohydrates. And there are so many sources! These starches are found in beans, legumes, nuts, and vegetables. When you focus on consuming vegetables as a

**MILLET:** High in protein, millet is popular around the world for humans, but in the United States it's mainly used for bird food—they're getting a great meal out in the bird feeder! Millet is gluten-free and naturally alkaline, with significant amounts of iron, lecithin, and choline, which help to keep cholesterol down.

**OATS:** A great source of natural oils, oats lower cholesterol and are high in fiber. Used to stabilize blood sugar levels, oats also improve stress resistance and are high in protein.

**QUINOA:** The only grain that is a complete protein, quinoa is good for vegetarians. A good source of iron, vitamins $B_3$ and $B_6$, and phosphorus, this small grain is easy to digest and supports the kidneys. Gluten-free and quick cooking, quinoa should be rinsed in three changes of water due to a naturally occurring *saponin,* which can cause it to taste bitter.

**RICE:** With hundreds of varieties to choose from, rice offers protein, fiber, calcium, iron, B vitamins, and zinc. Plus, it's gluten-free. Used in traditional Chinese medicine to promote good digestion, rice is also used to relieve depression, stop diarrhea, and support the spleen, pancreas, and stomach.

**RYE:** Used to boost the glandular system and support liver function, rye has a low gluten content. It's rich in protein, lysine, fiber, vitamins $B_6$ and E, calcium, copper, folate, and iron. Toasting the grains in a dry skillet and then boiling them as instructed brings out their delicious nutty flavor.

**SPELT BERRIES AND FLOUR:** Tolerated by many people who are allergic to wheat, spelt flour is a wonderful replacement for wheat in baking and has more amino acids, protein, minerals, and B vitamins than wheat. Helpful for blood clotting and boosting the immune system, it contains fiber, iron, copper, and phytochemicals.

main source of complex and simple carbohydrates, you will feel better because you are also getting higher amounts of phytonutrients, antioxidants, vitamins, and minerals. These are the powerful ingredients that we need the most in order to detox and heal from a lifetime of processed foods.

## WHOLE GRAIN COOKING MADE EASY

Americans have forgotten how to cook. The tradition of preparing food together and gathering for a meal has been lost in many households, unless you count the frantic scramble of holiday feasts. Even then, most of the cooking is left to a few individuals, usually women, who take the burden of cooking meals as just that: a burden. Food is a vital, living part of life and families. With a little planning and practice, home-cooked meals can become a regular source of connection and joy. When you make your own food, you know what you're getting—there's no guessing about what ingredients you might be consuming. The fresh foods you use and the nourishment you'll derive from your healthful choices will show up as increased energy, health, and vitality. To make real changes in your body and diet, you need knowledge and you need to take action. So get cookin'! Cooking whole grains can be really simple with a few tips and a little practice. Follow these simple steps using the "Cooking Whole Grains" chart on page 125 for great grains every time.

- Pour the indicated amount of liquid into a small or medium pot and bring to a boil.

- Add the grain with a pinch of salt, stir well to rid the grain of any clumps, and return to a boil for 2 minutes.

- Cover the pot with a tight-fitting lid and turn the heat down as low as possible, to bring the liquid to a simmer. Do not stir or take the lid off, and cook for the indicated amount of time.

- The steam holes that appear toward the end of the cooking time are what really do the work—do not stir to disturb these steam vents. By simply turning off the heat and keeping the lid on, the grain will continue to cook and steam for at least 5 more minutes.

- Cook once, eat thrice. Make a triple portion of your favorite grain and keep it in the refrigerator in an airtight container. Reuse over the next few days in soups, as side dishes with vegetables, mixed with beans, or even as a reheated breakfast cereal with fruit and nuts.
- Try thermos grains: Combine the indicated amount of grain and boiling water in a wide-mouthed thermos, stir well to break up any clumps, and seal the lid tightly. Leave undisturbed overnight. The next morning, the grain will be ready for breakfast, or as a quick lunch or snack for the day.

## Cooking Whole Grains

| GRAINS, DRY (1 CUP) | WATER OR BROTH | COOKING TIME | YIELD |
|---|---|---|---|
| Amaranth | 2½ cups | 20–30 minutes | 2 cups |
| Barley, hulled | 3 cups | 1½ hours | 3½ cups |
| Barley, pearled | 2½ cups | 1 hour | 1¼ cups |
| Cornmeal (polenta) | 3 cups | 20 minutes | 3 cups |
| Millet | 2½–3 cups | 30 minutes | 4 cups |
| Oats, rolled | 3 cups | 30 minutes | 4 cups |
| Oats, whole groats | 3 cups | 1–1½ hours | 2½ cups |
| Quinoa | 2 cups | 20 minutes | 2¾ cups |
| Rice, brown (long) | 2½ cups | 1 hour | 2½ cups |
| Rye berries | 3 cups | 2–2½ hours | 3 cups |
| Spelt berries | 3 cups | 2–2½ hours | 3 cups |
| Wheat, whole groats | 2½ cups | 35–50 minutes | 3 cups |

# STRESS LESSEN
## Movies to Get You Cookin'

Sometimes one of the best ways to relax is to totally "veg out," as my mom likes to say. Watching a good movie with a cup of tea can make all the stress just melt away. And some movies are inspirational in their content and can get us motivated to try new things in our lives. Some of my all-time favorite movies are about food. Check these out and see if you become as excited to get cooking as I do!

- *Babette's Feast:* A French chef is saved by two sisters in a remote Danish village, and to thank them for their kindness, she prepares an incredible feast of thanks and forgiveness.

- *Big Night:* Two Italian brothers try to make their restaurant a success in America with one last-ditch dinner party for reporters and friends.

- *Chocolat:* A young woman feeds homemade chocolates, love, and passion to her fellow townspeople.

- *Eat Drink Man Woman:* The ingredients of life are examined in this lovely, funny Chinese film about a retired chef and his three daughters who are forced to come home every week for a family dinner.

- *Like Water for Chocolate:* The history of a Mexican family is told through menus, a cookbook, and feasts.

- *Tampopo:* The first Japanese noodle western! A young widow is assisted by a mysterious truck driver to set up the perfect fast-food noodle shop. Hilarity ensues.

# MENTAL DETOX
## Living a Whole Life

No, "whole life" isn't just an insurance package—it's a bigger way to look at detoxification and vibrant, healthy living. Understanding where your food comes from means more than just the name of the grocery store where you buy your lettuce and noodles. Discovering the story behind the purchases you make opens up the world so that you can understand your power in the world—that *what you buy and eat matters*. Do you know in what country and under what conditions your food was grown or manufactured? Were the people or animals who worked to produce your food treated well? How many hands, from beginning to end, carried your food before it got to your table? How many ingredients, chemicals, or processes were involved in bringing one strawberry to your plate in winter? Your power as a consumer is strong, especially when you make well-informed decisions about how you will spend your food dollars.

**Exercise:** Choose one of your favorite foods and do some research: Where did your food come from? How was it grown? Use the Internet, call the toll-free number on the package, and read up on agricultural practices used in the country of origin. Since being a citizen is so closely linked with being a consumer, do your patriotic duty and get to know your food. Understanding how the food you eat went from the farm, to the supermarket, to your table will help you to better understand the whole world.

# CHAPTER 9

# Too Much of a Good Thing?

## Week 6: Finding a Balance with Protein
## Nutritional Issue: Protein Quantity

Most Americans eat too much protein, mainly because our diet is so high in animal meats and dairy products. According to the USDA, in 2000 annual meat consumption (red meat, poultry, and fish) reached 195 pounds per person, which is an increase of 57 pounds per person since the 1950s. It is recommended that men eat between 30 to 60 grams of protein a day, while women need between 25 and 50 grams of protein a day. Most Americans eat closer to 100 to 120 grams of protein per day, which just puts too much stress on the body.

We need protein for cell growth and maintenance. But protein cannot be stored in the body, so we have to take it in through our diets. Most Americans hold the false belief that protein comes only from meat and dairy sources, and then they overindulge in these food groups. Recent fad diets, like the Atkins diet and the Zone diet, have only encouraged our overconsumption of animal-based proteins, much to the detriment of our overall health. High-protein diets have been linked to certain cancers, osteoporosis, asthma, constipation, and migraine headaches.

During Morgan's fast-food-only month, he ate an unusual amount of animal protein. Hamburgers, cheeseburgers, bacon, breaded and fried chicken, milk, and eggs were in almost every meal he had. This overload of animal proteins, coupled with how overprocessed these foods were, had a toxic effect on his body. He was sluggish, he was depressed, and his liver became filled with fat.

Learning how much protein you need is an important part of detoxifying and remaining healthy and strong. Fortunately, our bodies give off clear signs when we are consuming too much—or too little—protein. Some people who are not getting enough protein have strong sugar and sweet cravings, are not able to concentrate, feel fatigued and spacey, are anemic, or have hair loss or unhealthy facial coloring. Too much protein can cause symptoms like low energy, constipation, tight or stiff joints, kidney disease, stress, bad body odor and bad breath, dehydration, and weight gain. Determining how much protein is best for you takes some self-awareness. How physical is your daily life and job? Are you pregnant or lactating? Do you feel well now, given how much protein is in your diet? Learning to trust your body and its messages is very important. Allow yourself to experiment some with how much and what kind of protein you include in your diet, and don't worry: It would be virtually impossible for anyone on the Standard American Diet to become protein deficient.

Part of the reason we're overdosing on protein is the problem with serving sizes (or lack thereof) in this country. Think back to the last time you ate a piece of meat or chicken. How big was it? This is an important question to ask, as we're routinely given huge portions (did the last steak you ordered cover the whole plate?). The American Dietetic Association has created some helpful visual comparisons so we can judge whether we are getting a reasonably sized portion or not. The average serving size of meat protein should be about the size of a deck of cards, not a roulette wheel. A serving of cheese should be the size of a domino, and a burrito the size of a bar of soap—not a torpedo. I know, I know. It is tough to eat less when all you're offered is too much. Most of us were trained to clean our plates, so eating in restaurants poses a portion-size dilemma: Do I eat only what my body needs or do I eat it all?

The current trend of high-protein, low-carbohydrate diets is potentially dangerous for other important reasons related to detoxification. The main organs involved in protein metabolism are the kidneys and liver. Over time, a diet high in protein may overtax these organs. People with liver diseases, diabetes, or alcoholism should be aware that digesting high amounts of protein requires more energy and a higher level of functioning than their already impaired organs can handle. But you don't have to be ill to benefit from finding nonanimal sources of protein. By mixing it up protein-wise, you'll be doing a better job of balancing your diet in ways that will help your metabolic systems function more efficiently and process protein with greater ease.

High-protein diets also concern health officials because they lower the pH balance of the blood. When you consume lots of protein and very little carbohydrates, you are not giving your body the sugars it needs to create glucose, which is the number one source of energy in our blood. When your blood sugar is low, your body must find an alternative source of energy, so it will use fat, instead of sugar, as a source of fuel. When fat is converted to fuel under these circumstances, it produces acidic particles known as ketones in a process that is called ketosis. The danger with ketosis is that it floods the blood with too many acids. No one yet knows for sure what impact this has on long-term health, but as with any kind of extreme dieting, it is wise to be cautious when you are eating in a way that alters your metabolism so dramatically. Being in a constant state of ketosis puts your body in a state of imbalance, and we know the body is happiest and healthiest when it's balanced.

Ketosis aside, most people who take on a high-protein diet in order to lose weight have trouble maintaining their weight loss. A report in the *New England Journal of Medicine* that tracked dieters on high-protein regimes noted that many regained their weight after 6 months and that most were unable to sustain weight loss after this. Additionally, high-protein diets tend to focus on controlling the intake of complex carbohydrates so strictly that even vegetables and fruits become restricted, which means that high-protein dieters run the risk of serious nutrient deficiencies since they don't have access to the vitamins and minerals found in these foods. Contrary to this theory, I encourage anyone eating meats to greatly increase his or her consumption of vegetables, especially leafy greens, to provide antioxidants, fiber, and slow-burning complex carbohydrates to complement and balance the intake of animal proteins.

Why do I recommend this? Our bodies have simply not evolved as quickly as our modern society has, and so our contemporary eating habits are out of sync with our biology. In the last 100 years, modern agriculture has changed the way we eat, refrigeration has changed the seasonal foods we have access to, and global transportation has opened up a world of cuisines and products to us. Imagine, in less than six generations, we've gone from eating local, seasonal, organically produced foods to a diet that is high in processed foods that are shipped in from all corners of the globe. In short, we can have anything we want to eat whenever we want it. Now we can eat strawberries in the middle of winter and tomatoes (or at least red objects that look like tomatoes) all year round. Even meat, which is now scientifically raised and fed with processed grains, is available anytime. Yet our bodies are still wired to respond to the limited choices offered by each season and actually suffer (like a child who eats too much cake at her birthday party) from the excess and convenience of modern, "seasonless" bounty.

## THE TOXIC LINKS IN THE PROTEIN FOOD CHAIN

The higher up on the food chain you eat, the more toxins, pesticides, and pollutants you are bringing into your body. The Environmental Protection Agency (EPA) admits that "nearly all fish and shellfish contain traces of mercury." Pollutants build up in the tissues of smaller animals, which are then eaten by larger animals, which are finally eaten by the animal at the top of the food chain—which is us humans. These toxins become more concentrated the higher up on the food chain you eat. For example, a small fish is eaten by a medium-size fish, which is eaten by a larger fish, which is eaten by you. Not only are you eating the fish, but you're eating all the fat-soluble toxins and pollutants that were lurking around in the small and medium-size fish. The toxins are passed upward, concentrating and increasing, until they reach dangerous proportions in the larger predatory fish.

## Something's Fishy

Major warnings are being issued more regularly now about the toxins found in fish. In the past decade, the number of U.S. states issuing warnings against eating fish because of mercury poisoning jumped from 27 to 45. Over the same period, the number of mercury-related "Fish Consumption Advisories" issued more than doubled (899 to 2,362). Farm-raised fish are generally fed a fish meal made from smaller, ground-up fish, while wild fish tend to eat a larger variety of foods found lower down the food chain. In addition, farm-raised fish are also treated with antibiotics to fend off the germs inherent in a fish-farm setting, and they're given hormones to make them grow bigger faster.

The EPA recommends that women of childbearing age and children avoid shark, swordfish, king mackerel, or tilefish because they contain high levels of mercury. While this recommendation makes sense, further recommendations for other types of fish seem contradictory. The EPA makes the recommendation that it is safe to eat two average-size meals a week of shrimp, canned light tuna, salmon, pollack, and catfish, which are lower in methyl mercury, and one meal of tuna steak per week. Methyl mercury is considered the most toxic form of mercury. Exposures to very small amounts can result in devastating neurological damage and death. If a mercury thermometer breaks, the air in the room can reach contamination levels quickly. This is dangerous stuff.

Extreme levels of PCBs, a known carcinogen, have been found in farm-raised salmon. In addition, traces of industrial-grade fire retardant have been found in farm-raised and wild salmon around the world. PBDEs, which are chemicals found in fire retardants, can harm neurological development and function in babies and young children—just like mercury and PCBs. Approximately 10 percent of U.S. women have mercury levels within one-tenth of hazardous levels. It is important to consider this statistic in light of the fact that the bulk of our exposure to mercury in the United States is through our consumption of fish.

To decrease the amount of contamination, choose a cooking method that allows most of the fat to drip away from the fish during the cooking process. Broiling and baking are better than frying. However, no cooking method will reduce the amount of methyl mercury, which is evenly distributed throughout the fish's tissues and meat. Experts recommend avoiding all of the cooking oils and drippings from cooked fish: That's how toxic this stuff is.

In truth, the toxicity of some of these chemicals isn't fully understood yet. However, the impact on our food supply is obvious—the more animal products we eat, the more toxins we are taking into our bodies. These chemicals leach out of their intended products and have been turning up everywhere—in our food, in dust samples, even in women's breast milk. Contaminants such as PCBs are fat-soluble and collect in the fatty tissue and skin of the fish.

## I'D BE A MAD COW, TOO

Meat and poultry are not off the hook in this discussion. While the shocking drama of mad cow disease played itself out in Europe, American meat producers scrambled to present our meat supply as safe and untainted. However, many of the same suspect production steps are still used in the United States, and factory farming on a huge scale continues to contribute to the problem. The globalization of meat production has created an atmosphere where meat and chicken can be processed in ways that add substantial water content to the final product. By adding salt, sugar, flavorings, gums, and additives, which may not appear on the label, meat can be sold at a greater price—just because of the sheer weight of these added "bonuses."

Global meat production and transportation has made it more difficult to know where and how our food is produced. Processing practices in developing countries in Asia and South America may have lower standards than their U.S. counterparts. A greater demand for cheaper foods has led to a worldwide consolidation of animal raising and food production, causing intensification of speed and quantity—while quality and safety suffer. This has all led to a system that promotes animal suffering, too, as they are packed into huge factories that are rife with disease, tainted food, and other health risks. These animals need drugs and hormones to make them grow bigger and antibiotics to keep rampant infection at bay.

The discovery of antibiotics is one of the greatest in human history. Our civilization surely wouldn't have developed so far if we had continued to be at risk of major widespread infections. However, now we're beginning to suffer the effects of way too much of a good thing. Seventy percent of all antibiotics used in America today are fed to livestock, and the residue is beginning to show up in rivers, streams, and soil near factory farms. The residues of these drugs are carried through our food and onto our plates, creating a constant stream of medication into our bodies. The results of these abuses have been the rise of untreatable strains of bacteria and "super bugs." These are stronger than our own immune systems or the best weaponry of our pharmaceutical industries, which are reluctant to spend the time and money to develop new and stronger antibiotics.

Pesticides and herbicides are a necessary part of the mono-cropping that is indicative of modern agriculture. Hundreds of acres of a single variety of plant are more prone to disease and infestation than mixed crops. As consumers, we are not only buying a food product, we are buying into a structure that uses billions of tons of poisons and drugs to keep this unsustainable system propped up. And we're paying the price for it, not only with our wallets, but with our health.

## THE DAIRY DILEMMA

Cow's milk is probably the most aggressively marketed food product in this country. Just pick up a magazine and there you'll find the celebrity of the day smiling with a milk moustache and the tagline "Milk: It Does a Body Good." Because of this aggressive marketing, most of us think that milk and/or dairy products are an essential food group. If you believe this, you are wrong. There is nothing essential (including calcium) in cow's milk or other dairy products that we can't get—in better form—from plant-based sources.

The milk industry (in conjunction with the U.S. Government) tells us that we should all drink three glasses a day for strong bones and healthy teeth. We're also told that milk is a great source of protein. What they're not telling you is that drinking this much milk—especially in conjunction with a high-protein diet—can actually cause our bodies to lose calcium!

Calcium, which is available in the blood in trace amounts, is necessary for blood clotting, muscle contraction, heartbeat maintenance, and healthy nerve function. Roughly 99 percent of the calcium in our bodies (about 3 pounds' worth) is stored in our bones and teeth, which rely on it for their strength. When it is needed, calcium is released from our bones into our blood.

So what happens when we follow the government's guidelines and we drink three glasses of milk a day, on top of eating too much animal protein? A high-protein diet, especially one built around animal products, makes our blood acidic, which is a condition the body tries to fix by pulling calcium (which is an alkaline mineral) from the bones. This is particularly a cause for concern with American women, who eat twice the amount of recommended daily protein. Once calcium is leeched from the bones, it leaves the body for good, via urine. This, surely, can lead to osteoporosis. Research shows that the nations with the highest calcium intake from dairy consumption have the highest rates of osteoporosis and hip fracture, while there are fewer such fractures in populations where dairy intake is low.

The truth is calcium is calcium (just as protein is protein). We can get calcium from plant sources in a form that doesn't disturb our blood pH levels and, consequently, allows our bodies to store the calcium more efficiently. Some research suggests that vegetarians—and vegans in particular (who eat no dairy)—enjoy diets rich in both protein and calcium but without the attendant blood acidity of their meat-eating counterparts and so, as a group, have better bone health.

Aside from the problems that calcium derived from cow's milk may cause to our bones, there are other problems with dairy as a source of protein and calcium. Milk is the most common cause of food allergies. Millions of people in this country have trouble digesting milk products because of the proteins or sugars found in milk. But our problems with lactose digestion shouldn't surprise us. Nutritional anthropologists believe that our earliest ancestors met all of their calcium needs by eating wild plant foods, and even had a higher level of calcium intake than we do now. Because humans didn't consume dairy products just 10,000 years ago, it makes sense to these scientists that our bodies would still have trouble processing this kind of food. Our bodies simply haven't evolved in keeping with the cultural pressure we're under to consume milk.

An overreliance on cow's milk in children can lead to anemia. This is because milk is low in iron, and kids who drink a lot of it may crowd iron-rich foods out of their diets. Cow's milk has also been linked to colic and ear infections in infants. Kids who drink a lot of milk through adolescence are also at greater risk for developing type 2 diabetes. The fat content in milk rates second only to that in beef (almost half the calories in milk are from fat) and has been linked to heart disease. For women who consume milk, the risk of osteoporosis, which I've already discussed, should be a serious concern, so too the link of milk consumption to ovarian cancer.

Consider the case of my client Paul, who missed eating dairy. Having been lactose intolerant for most of his life, he would still crave and eat milk, cheese, and butter occasionally. Drinking Lactaid-brand milks and swallowing special enzymes before cheesy meals helped him to digest the dairy, at least most of the time. During a session, Paul told me about a recent day when he had eaten a hearty amount of cheese for lunch on the same day he had a big bowl of cereal with milk. He described his stomach as "a pretzel, tied in knots" and said that he could feel how hard his body was working to try to digest the cheese. This realization was a real breakthrough. When you decide to detoxify your body, it's important that your organs and tissues are cared for properly. Since your digestive system is really the base of your overall health, stressing the intestines by forcing them to digest foods that are difficult for them causes the body to break down. When the digestive system isn't working, it can't draw out nutrients, provide the body with energy, or eliminate wastes properly. Paul realized that when he ate cheese, he was compromising his health in major ways.

If all of these facts aren't enough to give you pause before you reach for that glass of milk, there is also the problem of production. Cows in the United States are routinely given recombinant Bovine Growth Hormone (rBGH), which is meant to increase milk production in a country that is already producing and promoting too much milk. Many believe rBGH poses serious health risks for consumers (including raising antibiotic residue levels in milk). There are so many chemicals in our milk supply that *Washington Post* columnist Colman McCarthy remarked that it should be sold by prescription only.

If you do use cow's milk in your diet, you should buy only organic milk, in order to be ensured that the milk you are drinking is hormone- and antibiotic-free.

In 2001, Americans consumed 30 pounds of cheese per person, eight times more than they did in 1909 and more than twice as much as they did in 1975. Demand for time-saving convenience foods is a major force behind this growth in cheese consumption. Dairy-free cheeses, which are lower in fat and have no cholesterol, are improving in quality and can work for sandwiches and recipes when the craving strikes you. However, I recommend staying away from these highly processed cheese substitutes during your detox, as they are still far away from a whole food.

## Dangers in Our Food Supply

When I began working as a chef in New York City, I spent 6 hours a day, for 5 days in a row, sitting in a dingy basement classroom with 50 other food service workers. We were there to be educated on the finer points of safe food handling and to earn certification from the city. On the first morning our instructor, a precise, Caribbean-born gentleman, walked to the front of the classroom at exactly 9:00 A.M. and declared loudly, "You are ALL potential murderers!" He held our close attention for the next 5 days.

A former health inspector for the city, our teacher told us incredible stories of grime, filth, and illness found in the best and worst of New York's restaurants. We learned new words like *Campylobacter* and *Listeria*—words that strike fear into the heart of any food worker, and anguish into the hearts of parents and doctors across America. These are diseases that kill, and they come to us on our dinner plates.

The Centers for Disease Control (CDC) report that contaminated foods cause more than 70 million illnesses, 325,000 hospitalizations, and more than 5,000 deaths per year in America. Products containing dangerous bacteria range from apple juice to chicken sandwiches, but because fecal contamination is most often the cause, meat and poultry products are the main source of concern. In 2002, more than 60 million pounds of meat and poultry products were recalled by the USDA and CDC. Unfortunately, most of these massive recalls happen only after illness has been detected, or worse, after consumers have died.

Sanitation in the raising and manufacturing of these products is the main culprit of contamination. Large-scale meat-processing facilities are under pressure to produce more product faster, and sanitation measures suffer as a result. Fly and roach infestations, fecal contamination, outdated water systems, and a flawed inspection system have created a dangerous environment in our modern food supply. The General Accounting Office (GAO) found that even when processing plants are cited for unsafe or unsanitary conditions, they are allowed to continue operating.

The major pathogens that cause food-borne illness are familiar to most of America, and the symptoms are similar in most cases: diarrhea, abdominal pain, and fever. *Campylobacter* is present in more than 50 percent of the raw chicken sold in the United States. *Salmonella* is found in undercooked and raw eggs, poultry, pork, and beef. *E. coli* is most often found in ground beef. *Listeria* has been found in hot dogs, lunch and deli meats, juices, soft cheeses, and smoked seafood. Those with weakened immune systems, including the young and elderly, are especially at risk of contracting illnesses caused by these bugs.

Food irradiation was originally touted as the answer to all of our fears about food-borne illness when it was introduced more than 30 years ago. It has since been the focus of a lot of controversy, with several medical studies claiming that the process induces a chemical reaction in foods that makes them carcinogenic. In Europe the process is banned, except for treating spices and dried herbs. In the United States, the process has been used on a variety of meats, and in 2002, irradiated meat was allowed for use in the national school lunch program. During irradiation, meats are exposed to gamma rays, or electron beams, that kill harmful bacteria, insects, and parasites. However, irradiation also creates free radicals in the meat that contribute to disease and aging. Food irradiation is sold to us as a necessary technology, given the poor sanitary conditions that factory-farmed animals are raised in and the questionable manufacturing practices of meat suppliers. But this is just replacing one health risk with another. Consumer advocate groups are working to encourage livestock producers and meat manufacturers to make changes that will provide healthier living conditions for the animals and healthier processing procedures for their products.

People often ask me where I get my calcium if I don't eat dairy products. There are plenty of natural, delicious vegetable sources of calcium that also provide your body with the benefits of antioxidants, fiber, and minerals.

The Dietary Reference Intakes (DRIs) for calcium are 500 milligrams per day for children 1 to 3 years old; 800 milligrams per day for children 4 to 8 years old; 1,300 milligrams per day for adolescents and teenagers (9- to 18-year-olds); and 1,000 to 1,200 milligrams per day for those of us over 19. There are tremendous ways to get calcium from nondiary sources. Bear in mind that a cup of cow's milk provides 290 to 300 milligrams of calcium and compare this with the items listed in "Nondairy Sources of Calcium" on page 140.

Fortunately, it is easy to make substitutions for milk in baking and cooking, too. Milk can be replaced easily with an equal amount of water or fruit juice. (For example, substitute 1 cup milk with 1 cup water.)

There are many replacement foods that are available in most grocery stores, and more cookbooks and recipes designed for the lactose intolerant are popping up every year. Milks made from soy, rice, and nuts are commonly found in aseptic boxes, while you can make your own fresh nut milks very easily at home (see page 184 for a delicious recipe). Healthy oils can replace butter in cooking and baking, and I love drizzling extra-virgin olive oil on my air-popped popcorn. In the recipes section at the end of this book, you'll find several dairy-free recipes for favorite foods.

## HOW TO GET HEALTHY PROTEIN INTO YOUR DIET

When I talk with clients about protein, I have no agenda of wanting to make them eat the same way that I do, which is primarily free of animal products. I realize that everyone is different in terms of their lifestyle and basic body chemistry, and I respect people's traditional beliefs. There has long been a great debate between vegetarians and meat-eaters. I call it the great carnivore versus herbivore debate. People argue about tooth shape, intestinal tract length, and lactose intolerance. There are interesting points in these discussions, and exploring the realities of human evolution can shine a light on darker areas.

# Nondairy Sources of Calcium

| CALCIUM SOURCE | QUANTITY | CALCIUM (MILLIGRAMS) |
|---|---|---|
| Almonds | 1 oz (24 nuts) | 70 |
| Amaranth | 1 cup | 240 |
| Apricots | 3.5 oz | 67 |
| Beans, black | 1 cup | 120 |
| Beans, northern | 1 cup | 160 |
| Beet greens | 1 cup | 150–180 |
| Blackstrap molasses | 1 Tbsp | 175 |
| Bok choy | 1 cup | 158–200 |
| Breast milk, human | 3 oz | 33 |
| Broccoli | 1 cup | 160–180 |
| Collard greens | 1 cup | 225–300 |
| Dandelion greens | 1 cup | 140 |
| Dulse (sea vegetable) | 1 cup | 567 |
| Figs, dried | 5 figs | 135 |
| Kale | 1 cup | 180–200 |
| Kelp/kombu | 1 cup | 305 |
| Rhubarb | 1 cup | 250–360 |
| Sesame seeds (unhulled) | 1 oz | 381 |
| Soy milk (enriched) | 1 cup | 350 |
| Spinach | 1 cup | 175–244 |
| Tempeh | 1 cup | 150 |
| Tofu | 4 oz | 145–258 |
| Wakame (sea vegetable) | 1 cup | 520 |
| Yogurt | 1 cup | 440–490 |

When comparing a serious carnivore, like a dog or tiger, to a human being, some basic differences in physiology show up. A carnivore has sharp incisors, knifelike teeth for cutting and tearing flesh. An herbivore, like a cow, has flat molars, which are good for chewing fibrous greens and plant matter. Human beings have mostly molars, and our intestinal tract is long, curling, and twisted, much like that of cows and other herbivores. Heavier animal proteins take longer to digest and may get stuck and decay in our intestines. Men with diets that are high in meat are four times more likely to get colon cancer than vegetarians, according to Edward Giovannucci, professor of medicine at Harvard Medical School.

Though we can certainly eat too much protein and too many refined carbohydrates, it's pretty much impossible to eat too many vegetables.

The food guide pyramid displays a thick, juicy slice of ham next to some eggs, but it doesn't focus on teaching that healthy protein can be obtained from various sources besides animal products. An important part of nontoxic protein menus is being sure to include a variety of sources. For protein to work in the body, all of the essential amino acids must be present. Our bodies are able to create *nonessential* amino acids from other proteins that we eat, but *essential* amino acids must be consumed from our food. For instance, both beans and brown rice are rich in protein, but both are lacking in one or more essential amino acids. By combining these two foods, you create a dish that provides your body with a wonderful high-protein meal. One cup of soybeans sautéed with quinoa will supply you with more than 40 grams of complete protein—and none of the cholesterol or saturated fat that animal meats have.

Most nonanimal protein sources do not contain all of the necessary amino acids. This problem is easily solved by having several different foods together in one meal. By simply consuming a variety of whole grains, beans, and vegetables over the course of a day, you are sure to give your body everything it needs. Combining food in this way will also give you all of the components you need for proper protein absorption.

Soy-based foods are high in protein and easy to prepare. Every year, more products that offer soy's benefits line the shelves, but be aware that soy is one of the top 10 most allergenic foods. Signs of soy allergy include acne, anaphylaxis, gas, indigestion, cankers, conjunctivitis, dermatitis, and hives. However, tofu has been used in Traditional Chinese Medicine to neutralize toxins, so if you have no allergy to soy, it is a wonderful protein. When buying soy-based products, choose the foods that are labeled "organic" and "GMO-free." Most soybeans grown in the United States are genetically modified to withstand higher levels of pesticides and could be tainted with more harmful chemicals.

Detoxification by switching to vegetable sources of protein is simple. When you switch to a diet based on vegetable proteins, you automatically consume less antibiotics, cholesterol, saturated fats, nitrates, and hormones. The switch allows your body to calm down, clean out, and bulk up on healing nutrients, antioxidants, and phytonutrients. Cooking methods for protein can be less toxic if you avoid certain techniques. Charcoal grilling, frying, and broiling cause cancer-causing elements to form in the meat. Those criss-cross grill marks are pretty, but the effects on your body are not. Foods that are prepared by poaching, roasting, steaming, and stewing are much safer.

## STRESS LESSEN
### Aromatherapy in a Cup

Not only are fresh herbs great additions to meals, they are also invaluable aids when you're trying to relax, de-stress, and detox. A few simple herbs can be your "medicine chest" for natural anxiety relief, help with sleep, and general overall wellness. A simple tea can be made out of any of the following herbs. Place 1 teaspoon each of the herbs of your choice in a tea strainer and add a cup of boiling water. Allow to steep for 5 minutes, strain, and drink.

- Herbs and foods that soothe the nervous system: Chamomile, hops, passionflower, red clover, valerian
- Herbs and foods for easing blood pressure: Black cohosh, garlic, nettle, passionflower, Reishi mushrooms, Siberian ginseng, valerian
- Herbs and foods for relaxing before bedtime: Catnip, chamo-

# Plant Sources of Protein

| PROTEIN SOURCE | QUANTITY | PROTEIN (GRAMS) |
|---|---|---|
| Almonds | 1 oz (24 nuts) | 6.03 |
| Amaranth | 1 cup | 16 |
| Barley, pearled | 1 cup | 19.82 |
| Beans, refried (canned) | 1 cup | 13.83 |
| Beef, lean | 1 oz | 7 |
| Brazil nuts | 1 oz (7 nuts) | 4.07 |
| Buckwheat flour | 1 cup | 15.14 |
| Bulgur, dry | 1 cup | 17.21 |
| Cashew nuts | 1 oz (17 nuts) | 4.34 |
| Chickpeas/garbanzos | 1 cup cooked | 11.88 |
| Cornmeal | 1 cup | 11.7 |
| Couscous | 1 cup | 22.07 |
| Hazelnuts | 1 oz (19 nuts) | 4.24 |
| Lentils | 1 cup cooked | 17.86 |
| Macadamia nuts | 1 oz (11 nuts) | 2.21 |
| Peanuts | 1 oz | 6.71 |
| Pecans | 1 oz (19 nuts) | 2.6 |
| Quinoa | 1 cup | 22 |
| Soybeans | 1 cup cooked | 22.23 |
| Tempeh | 1 cup | 30 |
| Tofu | 1 cup | 20 |
| Walnuts | 1 oz (10 nuts) | 4.32 |
| Wheat flour, white | 1 cup | 12.36 |
| Wheat flour, whole | 1 cup | 16.44 |
| White beans | 1 cup cooked | 19.02 |

**NOTES:** 1 cup cooked beans or 2 eggs equals one 2- to 3-ounce serving of meat or poultry. One serving of lean or medium-fat meat contains 7 grams of protein.

mile, hops, lemon balm, passionflower, valerian, vervain, wild
lettuce

- Herbal tea for insomnia: Combine a teaspoon each of chamomile, lavender, lemon balm, passionflower, and valerian

# MENTAL DETOX
## Inner Strength, Inner Wisdom

We have been taught that protein is needed to make our bodies
strong and to repair damage, but what have we been taught about
how to heal our spirits and minds? Strength, above all, is valued in
today's modern world as the finest of characteristics. Don't let your
emotions get the best of you. Boys don't cry. You've got to hold on
and be strong. We may be paying a price for all of this rigid outer
strength that we are required to show to the world around us.
Gulping down emotions helps no one. Pressure to "shrug it off,"
"get over it," and "move on" without inconveniencing or embar-
rassing anyone with our emotions causes us to discount the very reality of our own feelings and experiences. In reality, opening up and
being honest about our fears and weaknesses may be one of the
strongest things we can do.

Exercise: Use a blank sheet of paper or a page in your journal
to write about your current fears. Write about your past fears also.
Are there fears from childhood that are still with you? Were you
afraid of the dark? Were you afraid of not being liked because your
parents told you there was something wrong with you? Were you
teased by other kids in school? Describe these fears in detail and
allow the hurt to fill up the page. Let the anger and hurt flow down
your arm, into your pen, and onto the page that can't talk back. Use
this exercise to see what your fears and weaknesses really are. Perhaps they are lingering voices from the past that, once recognized
for what they truly are, can no longer hurt you. See how your fears
have affected your life and choices throughout the years. What are
you holding on to from the past that is trapped in your body and
mind? See your fears melt onto the page and release their toxic hold
on you.

# CHAPTER 10

# Beyond Your Diet

## Week 7: Detoxing and the World around You Environmental Issues

Look around you. You'll see that the environment around us is constantly being polluted by noise, air pollution, garbage, toxic waste, and many kinds of toxins that poison our rivers, streams, lakes, and land. Just as toxic food poisons our bodies, these environmental toxins affect us, too.

In 2002, the Environmental Protection Agency (EPA) reported that mercury emissions, a powerful neurotoxin, had increased 10 percent, while lead levels were up 3 percent and dioxin levels up 5 percent. I share these statistics so you'll understand that, though you are detoxing your body by adjusting your diet, the world around you just hasn't caught up. But there are things you can do to mitigate the damage nonedible toxins have on you. And the key to doing this is to gain knowledge. By understanding your ability to create a detoxified home environment, you can protect yourself, your family, and, in part, the world around you, by making a commitment to live more cleanly.

## DETOXIFYING BEGINS AT HOME

One of the easiest ways to reduce our exposure to toxins is to really clean up our homes. For many people, the words *toxic* and *toxins* conjure up images of Chernobyl, Three Mile Island, and Superfund sites. But a surprising number of the most-harmful toxins ever created are found right in our own backyards, indeed in our very kitchens, bathrooms, and garages.

## PLASTIC'S NOT FANTASTIC

How much plastic (and I don't mean credit cards) is in your life? We are literally drowning in a sea of plastic, and this is not good news. Toys, food containers, plastic food wrap, appliances, and countless other items are made with plastics that contain petroleum, or oil, and innumerable other chemicals and toxins. And plastic isn't just in everything around us—it is in us, too, as the chemicals that make up plastic are constantly being leeched out of plastic and into the air and our food and water. Our lives are steeped in plastic because it is convenient (that word again) and relatively inexpensive. At least on the face of it. In an excellent article published on the Web site www.mindfully.org, Paul Goettlich points out that though plastic may seem cheap at first, no one is taking into account the money we have to spend to cope with all this "convenience." We pay municipal taxes to fund curbside recycling programs and to have all that plastic hauled away; we pay the cost for landfill space; and we pay the cost of incineration, which is the only way to truly destroy plastic, but which only produces more toxins. The ubiquitous use of plastic also increases our health costs, due to the health problems we all face from the toxins from plastic that enter our bodies when we eat them, drink them, or breathe them in.

Taking into account the "life cycle" of plastic forces us to rethink how wise it is to let it have a starring role in our convenience-oriented lifestyles. The truth is, plastics do stay with us forever—literally. They are absolutely nonbiodegradable, so every plastic that has ever been made is still with us. Unless, of course, it has been burned, which leads to a whole different issue regarding the toxins released in the lethal smoke this process creates. Fortunately for us (but unfortunately for our already beleaguered landscape), plastic production, for the long haul, simply isn't sustainable. More than 80 percent of the oil reserves discovered in North America have been depleted, and much of that oil goes toward the production of plastics. And landfills are filling up daily with mountains of plastic that will be with us for many years to come.

Every time you wear something that has plastic in it, sit on something that is made with plastic, or inhale the air in a room filled with plastics, you are ingesting plastic. Every time you eat or drink something served on or stored in plastic, you are ingesting the chemicals that make up that plastic.

Plastics are so easily ingested that the FDA (which calls plastics "food contact substances," just a nice way of saying "additives") has assumed for roughly 50 years that all plastics transfer toxins to the food they come in contact with. So why is it that we're just learning about this danger? Part of the problem is that the FDA has relied on the very manufacturers of plastics to test and control for the "migration" of toxins out of their products, and this has created a huge gap between our interests and the interests of the plastic makers. Fortunately for us, many public advocacy groups are beginning to focus intently on the health risks of exposure to plastic toxins, and because of these efforts, we now know that there are certain plastics that are worse than others. But this knowledge shouldn't mislead us: The truth is that it doesn't look like any type of plastic is actually "good," as all of them leech and release toxins when they come into contact with food.

The worst kind of plastic, in terms of toxicity, and for any use, but especially for use around food, is polyvinylchloride (or PVC). PVC is, on its own, quite rigid. But many chemicals are added to it to keep it soft and "flexible." All kinds of storage containers for food (including baby drinking cups, plates, and utensils) are made with PVCs. But most of us don't know that the chemicals that have been added to the PVC (they fill in the spaces between PVC molecules, therefore keeping them away from one another and preventing the PVC from becoming rigid) leak out of it constantly. This leaking becomes worse and worse over time.

We should be alarmed by this because research is showing that it isn't just high doses of PVC toxins that are harmful to us, but that even low doses that we take in over time can have serious consequences.

## The Effects of Plastic Toxins on the Body

Even extremely low doses of the toxins found in plastics (we're talking single digit—or lower—parts per trillion, or ppt) can tamper with the natural balance of the endocrine system. As Goettlich reminds us, these toxins are known as endocrine disruptors (EDs) and they "interfere with the production, release, transport, metabolism, binding, action, or elimination of natural hormones in the body responsible for maintaining internal balances and the regulation of developmental processes." This means that those who are at highest risk for endocrine dysfunction are those who are growing, and this population includes all children from conception to adulthood.

So think about what you have tucked away in your fridge, in your cabinets, and on your shelves. Anything that is stored in "disposable" plastic is becoming saturated with toxins while you read this. Now that I've given you the bad news, here's the really bad news:

All of these plastics (and this includes plastic wraps for food) really break down once they are heated. That's why it's very important not to reheat food in a plastic container or even on a plate with plastic wrap on top of it. When these plastic films get hot, they leak more and more toxic chemicals into our food.

Now that you are eating a healthier diet and have cut the toxins you ingest via your food supply, doesn't it only make sense to avoid putting other toxic chemicals into that food via the plate you serve it on? For the myriad reasons outlined above, I recommend that you switch as soon as possible to safer, more sustainable containers like those made of glass, ceramics, or nonreactive metals. By doing this, you will not only be protecting your own health, you'll be contributing to the greater well-being of the beautiful environment that surrounds us all.

## Bottled Water: Choose the Lesser Evil

Now that you're working to take in a minimum of 8 to 10 glasses of water a day, you're probably wondering how on earth you'll be able to do that without reaching for a plastic bottle of water. Since bottled water has become a staple in this country, you would be hard-pressed to avoid it at all times, but I urge you to try. Since plastic can't be entirely avoided, do try to make an effort to choose a less toxic kind of plastic bottle. Stay away from 1-gallon or larger plastic water containers unless they are labeled 2HDPE, since they may otherwise be made of PVC. Instead, purchase your drinking water in clear polyethylene or glass containers. Glass containers are the best option for drinking water, as they can be washed and reused almost indefinitely, and they don't leach any chemicals into the liquid. Refilling your own glass bottles at home for daily use is the cheapest option, and it's less harmful to the environment because it stops the need for throwaway plastic containers.

The safest plastic bottles and containers for storing food and liquid are:

■ Polypropylene: labeled "#5 PP"

■ High-density polyethylene: labeled "#2 HDPE"

■ Low-density polyethylene: labeled "#4 LDPE"

## SAFE POTS AND PANS

Now that you are putting beautiful, healing foods on your plate, how are you preparing them? Pots and pans come in a great variety of sizes, shapes, and materials. Aluminum cookware has gone out of favor, given the links that we know exist between aluminum and Alzheimer's disease. I advise avoiding using aluminum pans and one-use catering trays. Nonstick Teflon pans contain perfluorooctanoic acid (PFOA), a soaplike ingredient used in the manufacturing of nonstick kitchen skillets. PFOA is a fluorochemical that never breaks down and has been linked with birth defects per the EPA. The safest cooking pots and pans are those made out of stainless steel, cast iron, copper, clay, or glass.

# CHEMICALS IN OUR HOMES

Now that you've taken a look at what kinds of containers you're using for storing your food and also the pots, pans, and utensils that you use to prepare it, it's time to take a look at what kinds of cleaning products you have stowed under the kitchen sink, in the bathroom, and in the garage.

Although our bodies are designed to defend us against germs, bacteria, and allergens, they are hard-pressed to constantly fight off the damage brought on by industrially produced toxins. Our immune systems have enough to cope with without the added stress of these additional pollutants. Our bodies are already overtaxed coping with the poor Standard American Diet. They just don't have a fighting chance against the potent toxins that are lurking in the cleaning products we use every day.

In just the past few years, this has become glaringly obvious, as the incidences of diseases such as asthma and "sick building syndrome" (a newly coined phrase that describes the cluster of symptoms that people who live in dangerously compromised homes, or who work in toxic buildings, suffer from) have skyrocketed.

Because the symptoms of environmental toxicity are so varied, many of us get sick but go undiagnosed for years, because the source of our illness is just too hard to pin down. Asthma, headaches, memory loss, ringing in the ears, nausea, eczema, depression, chronic flulike symptoms, watery eyes, and exhaustion are all symptoms of environmental poisoning. But we can combat this by working to identify the products in our lives that may be contributing to our overall malaise.

Once we've identified the source of the environmental pollution that is making us sick, we can remove it from our lives and begin to detox from it. However, if you've been overexposed to one or several harmful chemical toxins, you will likely need the support of a medical professional to truly detox and regain your health.

In our attempts to get our clothes whiter than white and to keep our homes sparkling clean, we've brought powerful cleaning agents into our homes that simply shouldn't be there. Most of us don't know it, but many of the chemicals that are found in conventional household cleaning products are not regulated in any meaningful way as being safe for home use. What's more, many of these same chemicals are banned in our public workplaces, due to the acknowledgment of their harmfulness and the regulations that ban them, which the Occupational Health and Safety Administration (OSHA) has put into place!

We need to cut our exposure to harmful chemicals as much as possible in order to thrive and heal. The average American home uses and stores approximately 60 potentially hazardous household products at any given time. That translates into roughly 3 to 10 gallons of toxic chemicals and cleaners that are sitting around us sharing our most intimate environment. Many of these chemicals are unregulated by any government labeling laws, and we bring them into our homes without knowing that they may make us sick. Toxic chemicals are found in window, tile, drain, and carpet cleaners as well as in chlorine bleach, metal polishes, and weed killers. While these products may clean and brighten our homes, our bodies are coming into contact with these chemicals on a daily basis. In addition, our clothing, furniture, and even our children's toys may have been manufactured and processed using toxic materials.

These "everyday" toxins cause a whole host of physical problems, yet most of us don't make this simple connection. Common complaints that arise around the use of household cleaning products include chronic respiratory problems, rashes, fatigue, immune suppression, eye irritation, and headaches. Further, these chemicals have been linked with certain cancers and are known endocrine system disruptors. Some of the hazardous volatile organic compounds (VOCs) that are found in household products are toluene, styrene, xylenes, and trichloroethylene; these may be found in aerosol products, dry-cleaned clothing, paints, varnishes, glues, art supplies, cleaners, spot removers, floor waxes and polishes, and air fresheners.

## Household Cleaning Products: Toxins Galore

Most of us hate cleaning, so we turn to products that are aggressively marketed to us as—yet again—being convenient. We all know how horrible a task it is to clean the oven, so we all jump at the chance to grab a can of powerful oven cleaner that promises to do the work for us. What we fail to take into account is how harmful the fumes and chemicals that this kind of product releases are to our skin and respiratory systems. (Oven cleaner is particularly concerning as it releases such a high concentration of toxic fumes.) If we knew how harmful they are, we'd avoid them at all costs. In the case of cleaning your oven, I recommend putting a drip pan in the bottom of your oven. And wipe up spills as soon as they happen and before they become hardened and baked on to the oven. By taking care of spills when they happen, you can usually clean even heavy-duty appliances like your oven with just some water, soap, and a bit of elbow grease.

Do you have a jug of bleach under your sink? You might want to reconsider this. Chlorine, which is an active ingredient in bleach, is a potent toxin. When subjected to high heat, chlorine spawns dioxins, which are highly carcinogenic. Chlorine is also a component of the dangerous PCBs, or polychlorinated biphenyls, which continuously pollute our air and water. Instead of using cleaners (like bleach) that contain chlorine, try using more-natural cleansers. The following brands make excellent toxin-free cleansers: Earth Friendly, Citra-Solv, Bi-O-Kleen, and Seventh Generation. Also, by switching to unbleached toilet paper, paper towels, and coffee filters, you'll reduce the amount of dioxins that enter your home. There are also several natural approaches to maintaining clean swimming pools and hot tubs that don't rely on chlorine. Ask your local pool supply dealer for information on natural products.

What's truly scary about keeping these cleaning products in our homes is that, even when they are out of sight, tightly sealed, and seemingly well-contained, they are contributing to a very serious problem: indoor air pollution.

## INDOOR AIR POLLUTION

Many of us think that air pollution is a problem that happens only outdoors, especially in highly populated cities or near power plants, factories, or other environments that are dense with highly toxic emissions. But we're wildly mistaken about this. The EPA estimates that, on average, indoor air pollution is two to five times greater than outdoor air pollution! This fact should be of particular concern to all of us, as we spend anywhere from 50 to 90 percent of our time indoors, and most of that time is in our homes.

The Consumer Protection Agency (CPA) estimates that more than 150 chemicals found in the home are connected to allergies, birth defects, cancer, and psychological disorders.

But it's not just cleaning products that are toxic to us. Indoor air pollution may also be caused by several seemingly harmless products and furnishings. Many cushions on furniture are made from polyurethane plastic and are covered in acrylic, polyester, or polyvinyl chloride. Bookcases and furniture are often made from plywood and pressed particleboard, which are often treated with dangerous formaldehyde and may "off-gas" fumes for up to 5 years after they are manufactured. Carpets contain synthetic fibers, as well as formaldehyde and pesticides for mothproofing, and these toxins become airborne, too.

This kind of indoor air pollution is bad for us and worse for our kids. So how can you keep a clean home and still avoid these nasty, unseen pollutants? First, open your windows. To reduce the impact of indoor air pollutants, circulate fresh air through your house as often as possible by letting fresh air in by opening doors and windows or by using fans. If you are remodeling, ask your contractor to use low-VOC paints and stains, and avoid spray paint completely. Purchase furniture with untreated, whole wood frames and wool and cotton cushions whenever possible. Carpets may be sprayed with sealants that will keep fumes and off-gassing to a minimum, or you may choose to remove the carpeting and replace it with hardwood floors. Remember, your health is worth more than your carpeting. Keeping one or two green houseplants in several rooms of your home or office can remove some toxic chemicals from the air, and plants are a beautiful, natural source of fresh oxygen.

Many of us buy and use candles, believing that their lovely smells are freshening the air we breathe, when in fact most candles pollute the air. When buying candles, choose products made with vegetable oils such as soy or palm oil instead of petroleum waxes. Avoid candles that are scented with synthetic perfumes and try pure beeswax candles instead, which have a lovely faint honey scent, but which don't add unwanted fumes to your air. Wicks containing lead and other heavy metals can fuel a thin black smoke that is harmful and that throws off toxic residues that can quickly concentrate in the small spaces of our homes. Choose candles that have natural cotton or fabric wicks instead of metal ones.

## A Breath of Fresh Air

Ensuring that your home has clean air can go a long way in lightening the load of environmental toxins that your body has to combat and filter every day. There are several different air filters that promise to remove dust, mold, spores, and toxic fumes from the air. High tech and expensive air filtering systems have become big business—but buyer beware: in April 2005 *Consumer Reports* magazine released a review of ionizing air filters and found that several popular brands not only do a poor job of cleaning the air but that they also release potentially harmful amounts of ozone into your home's atmosphere. Instead of spending money on one of these questionable gadgets, just throw open your doors and windows and let the air outside circulate through your home. Also keep one or two green houseplants in each room because this will also help to keep the air in your home fresh and clean.

# A NATURALLY CLEAN HOME

Switching to safe, nontoxic cleaning products is an easy way to reduce the amount of pollution in your home. No law requires manufacturers of cleaning products to list ingredients on their labels or to test their products for safety. When you buy new cleaning products, look for manufacturers who list the ingredients on the label, and purchase cleansers that contain nonpetroleum-based surfactants, are chlorine- and phosphate-free, claim to be "nontoxic," and are biodegradable.

Natural home cleaning means using cleansers made with safe ingredients that are free of chlorine, ammonia, and chemicals. Cleansers made from vinegar, baking soda, water, herbs, essential oils, vegetable oils, lemon juice, and salt really work and do a fine job of keeping your home safe and clean. Essential oils like lavender, grapefruit seed, and tea tree oil can be used for antibacterial, antiviral, and antifungal cleansers. In her fantastic book *Better Basics for the Home,* Annie Berthold-Bond presents hundreds of easy formulas for homemade cleansers, deodorizers, lawn and garden care products, and even beauty aids. Switching to these homemade formulas is inexpensive and frees your home of unwanted chemicals. Seventh Generation, Dr. Bronner's, Earth Friendly Products, and Citrus Magic are some manufacturers that make a wide variety of household cleaning products that are safe and effective.

## NATURAL BEAUTY

The FDA regulates health and beauty products in the United States. However, this regulation has one glaring problem—the FDA is not legally empowered to require safety testing for the ingredients in our personal care products. According to a report by the Environmental Working Group (EWG), titled "Skin Deep," the FDA has testing information on only 11 percent of the 10,500 different ingredients found in our shampoos, face creams, and other beauty products. Not only is the evidence that these ingredients are safe sorely lacking, but the testing was conducted by a cosmetic industry board, not by an independent organization. More impor-

---

### Simple Homemade All-Purpose Cleaners

It's easy to mix up safe, effective, and inexpensive cleaners at home. Here are two of my favorites.

**HOMEMADE ALL-PURPOSE HOUSEHOLD CLEANER #1:** In a spray bottle, mix 2 tablespoons baking soda with 1 pint warm water. Add 1 tablespoon lemon juice or vinegar to cut grease. Spray, apply elbow grease, and wipe with a cloth.

**HOMEMADE ALL-PURPOSE HOUSEHOLD CLEANER #2:** Pour 1 pint club soda into a spray bottle. Spray, apply elbow grease, and wipe with a cloth.

---

tant, one out of every 120 of these common products contains ingredients identified as a "known or probable carcinogen." Several moisture creams and sunscreen products contain alpha and beta hydroxy acids, which, contrary to popular belief, can actually increase skin cancer risks.

The study estimates that the average American adult uses nine of these products a day and is exposed to about 126 different chemicals through this use. These chemicals, in small doses, may pose little threat. However, over time, in repeated doses, there can be a buildup of toxins in our skin and organs, which may lead to severe health problems. For example, some studies show that people with Alzheimer's disease have more aluminum than usual in their brains, and many antiperspirants contain aluminum.

More and more people are becoming allergic to their homes, offices, and the beauty and cleaning products they use every day. Environmental allergies cause fatigue, depression, headaches, and immune system dysfunction. I strongly urge my clients to scrutinize the labels on their cosmetics and personal care products. The easiest way to avoid toxic chemicals is to use products that are made from natural, plant-derived ingredients. A database has been compiled by EWG that lists the specific chemicals and hazards contained in more than 7,000 products; you can find it at www.ewg.org/reports/skindeep/.

## CLEAN CLOTHES

If your skin is sensitive to chemicals or you have experienced environmental allergies, be aware of your clothing. It's always around us, and it could be adding to our increased sensitivity. According to the U.S. Geological Survey, more than 60 pesticides with as much as 7 kilograms per hectare of herbicide and 5 kilograms per hectare of insecticide are sprayed on cotton crops grown in the United States. With more than 14 million acres of cotton being grown every year, which is then made into our clothing, it is inevitable that our skin comes into contact with these powerful toxins. By choosing clothes made from organic cotton, silk, or hemp, you will reduce this contact.

# STRESS LESSEN
## Lose the Clutter Instead of Losing Your Mind!

Detoxification means getting rid of the excess, negative aspects of living. This applies to both the chemical toxins stored in our bodies and the piles of junk stored in our homes. Is your dining room table covered in papers and boxes instead of being used for sitting and eating? Do you have to take out stacks of plastic containers from the cupboard to find some long-lost kitchen tool? Is your closet overflowing with old and rarely worn clothes that haven't seen the light of day in more than a year?

Cleaning out and lightening your load at home can help to calm your mind and focus your energies. Getting rid of a bunch of junk is very liberating! Clear out the old to make way for the new.

- Donate a large box of clothing to charity: Anything that you haven't worn in more than a year must go.
- Recycle any magazines that are more than 2 months old.
- Give away or recycle all plastic food containers. You may keep the ones that you use on a *weekly basis*. Otherwise, they have to go.
- Have a garage sale! Selling off your old stuff will bring in extra cash and free up space for a simplified life.

# MENTAL DETOX
## Nature's Healing Power

Sunny days, sweeping the clouds away indeed! Nature is the ultimate healing force—most of our prescription drugs are inspired by or extracted from natural sources, including plants, trees, and flowers. And exposing yourself to the calming wholeness of nature's gifts can bring relaxation, inner peace, and a sense of belonging. I've been called a tree hugger for good reason: When I'm sitting and communing quietly with nature, I feel a sense of love and happiness that I feel only when I'm outdoors in natural space. But all of us can benefit from spending more time in nature. Nancy Wells, an environmental psychologist at Cornell University in Ithaca, New York, has studied the effect of nature on children's ability to deal with stress. Her studies have found that rural children with access to outdoor greenery, as well as city kids with lots of houseplants in their homes, seem better able to handle stress and to focus on tasks than kids with no greenery in their lives. Not only are we relaxed by nature, but the sun's rays are needed to help our bodies create vitamin D, which allows the body to utilize and absorb calcium. In natural settings, most of us feel an increased sense of energy, well-being, and strength. Connecting with the natural world is an invaluable way to detox and rejuvenate. Plus it is free, easy, and powerful.

**Exercise:** On a scale of 1 to 10, with 1 being "terrible" and 10 being "fantastic," rate your overall feeling at this moment. Then go outside and choose a spot in a natural setting that is comfortable and attractive to you. This could be a local park, a botanical garden, a nature preserve—even a backyard or patio will work well. Spend 20 to 30 minutes exploring the area you have chosen. Feel the plants, trees, and grass as you wander through them. Smell the scents of the flowers and leaves. Listen to the sounds of the earth and wind. After the time has passed, check in and rate how you are feeling again. Has your mood improved? Are you more relaxed? Consider this improvement and remember that nature is always there for healing when you need it.

# CHAPTER 11

# Detoxing Your Life for Life

## Week 8: Committing to the Detox Lifestyle Changing Our Minds Means Changing Our Lives

Detoxification is a way of life, not just a diet. Just as what we eat builds up over time within our bodies, how we interact with the world around us can either fill us with toxins or open us up to healing. The progression from a toxic lifestyle to a healthy, disease-free life is all about learning how the world works, learning how your body works, and learning what choices you have available to you to create a world of health around you. When I began my own detox and began to pull myself out of the well of dis-ease and ill health I had fallen into, I reached out to the people around me, found information in my library, and spoke with alternative health experts for every bit of knowledge I could find. In short, I armed myself with the information I needed to make lasting and meaningful change, and I empowered myself by surrounding myself with nurturing and supportive people.

Learning that the foods I had come to rely on were actually the source of my misery was the first big step toward detoxing my life. Learning how to eat, grocery shop, and cook all over again was a challenge, but it was easier than being sick and miserable. Watching Morgan turn from a vibrant and healthy being into a sickly, exhausted person brought back memories of my own past health problems, and helping him with his detox reinforced for me how positive and life-affirming the journey to health is. Morgan's recovery and detoxification reminded me how important it is to build a community around yourself that is truly committed to you and your quest for a healthier way to live.

As I work with more and more clients, I experience their successes with a renewed appreciation for how unique we all are, in body and soul. And it confirms for me that we are all capable of actualizing true, meaningful change. Each of us can learn to take control of our health and become our own health advocates. After all, no one knows you better than you do!

Choosing healing, calming foods is the basis of this overall detoxification. Allowing the body time off from the powerful, dangerous junk foods that make up the Standard American Diet allows your body to heal and revitalize. But once your body is on the road to wellness, it is important to attend to the other aspects of your life that need detoxing, too.

# TAKE ACTION AND DETOX!

It's not enough to just put healthier food into your body. That's just the beginning. How, where, and when we eat is important, too. Sitting down to a meal is a great time to renew our spirits and collect our thoughts. It's also a great time to connect with others in a meaningful and relaxing ritualistic way.

## Mindless Eating and Awareness

Sitting and snacking are probably the two favorite all-American pastimes. Eating on the couch while sitting in front of the television set distracts us from the activity of eating and numbs our awareness as to what we are putting into our bodies. Turn off the television, pick up your plate, and relocate yourself to a peaceful and focused place to eat. By turning off the outside noise from the radio and television, we are able to focus on our meals and listen to our bodies while we eat. If we eat without distraction, we're much more likely to put nutritious foods into our bodies, and we're much more likely to hear our bodies when they are telling us they are full.

To facilitate this, I recommend that you begin to loosen the grip that television has on your life. Make a commitment that you'll get the noise of the media, advertisers, and shock jocks out of your head so that you are truly available to yourself and those around you at mealtime. When you turn off the television, which keeps your attention glued to an inanimate, "unreal" world, your senses will be freed to engage in the natural, real world that surrounds you.

Regardless of how well I eat, when I'm stressed out or unhappy in my work or my relationships, I still feel miserable. I feel terrible eating a beautiful bowl full of organic vegetables when I'm sitting in a messy living room with piles of unfinished business to attend to. The amount of stress that we encounter in our daily lives has a profound effect on our overall health. The human body is amazingly strong and resilient, but constant stress over time can compromise our immune systems and lead to toxic overload and eventual breakdown.

Everyone experiences stress in different ways and from different sources. Positive stress is actually good—it keeps us alert in times of danger, heightens our senses, and readies our bodies for action. However, constant negative stress, or distress, can lead to immune disorders, gastrointestinal problems, allergies, insomnia, depression, fatigue, sexual dysfunction, hair loss, and cardiovascular disease— wow! Sounds like these are good reasons to chill out! The key to understanding our stress is to understand the mind-body connection. We feel stress when we are unable to deal with change—but change is inevitable in life. Learning to *manage* stress and deal with change is the best way to minimize its negative effects on our lives and to reap the benefits of its positive aspects.

We even *stress-eat*. Picture this—you're overworked and not making as much money as you would like. You have no time to take care of yourself, and food seems more of a hassle than anything else.

Your head aches, your eyes are tired, and you have no energy. So you go to the drive-thru and grab some fast food to save time and effort. This fast food fills your stomach with excess sugar, caffeine, and food additives, which might offer a short-term sense of well-being (your stomach is full) but actually stress your body more. Sadly, this is the typical American way of life. We're so chronically stressed out that we stop loving and caring for ourselves: We treat our pets better than this! But it's not just our eating habits that erode. We engage in other activities that are toxic to our lives as well. For many of us, shopping becomes a form of "retail therapy," a misguided way to show ourselves love and care. But this only adds to the toxicity of our lives by driving us into financial debt and clogging our homes with more junk we just don't need. And it perpetuates the cycle we desperately need to break: We work more just to pay the bills, we lose more sleep, we continue to eat on the fly, and so on. It's all related: The convenient life, as it turns out, is conveniently killing us.

So what can we do to deal with change and lessen the effects of stress? Building a strong body is the first line of defense and will give you the resilience you need to deal with stress in healthy ways.

When we're under stress, our bodies react with a flurry of biochemical activity. Neurotransmitters get activated, hormones are released, and nutrient metabolism slows down. Some of our bodily systems get ramped up: Our hearts start to pump faster, and so our blood pressure goes up. Some of our systems slow down, such as our gastrointestinal processes. All these things occur because the body is being given the message that it is going to need to "take action" in order to cope with the stress it is experiencing. But in our modern lives, we're not usually confronting a form of physical stress: We're more often suffering psychic stress, and so we're not using our bodies (which are now in a heightened state of readiness) to tackle the problem. Our bodies, then, are left with the toxic fallout from the activated but unused "fight or flight" response. As the physiological by-products of this stress response continue to circulate, our bodies become run down. Regular exercise, in this age of nonphysical stress, is the best way to flush these toxins out of our systems and give our bodies a rest from being so "stressed" out.

Being sedentary is, sadly, one of the core problems with the modern American lifestyle. Along with eating a balanced, wholesome diet, we need to exercise regularly in order to experience true health. We all know that diet alone will not help us shed weight effectively and that exercise is crucial to making this happen. What we don't know is that regular exercise is also needed to maintain health and to ensure longevity. Study after study has shown that exercising is key to preventing a huge host of illnesses. As Ernest Randolfi, Ph.D., points out on his excellent Web site, OptimalHealthConcepts.com, "Inactivity should be considered a dis-ease state." He also points out that most of us complain that we just don't have time to exercise. Why is it, then, that "a high percentage of CEOs of Fortune 500 companies indicate that they exercise on a regular basis" and that "even the president of our country seems to find time in his busy schedule to jog and play golf." These achievers have learned that the only way to meet stress head-on and in a healthy way is to get moving! It is time we all learned to do the same.

## MOVING FOR HEALTH

My client, Kris, was having a hard time getting excited about exercise—there were always reasons and excuses to avoid getting active, and she lived in a very hot part of the country. We talked about how she might tap into her motivation and also what different types of exercise to try: Yoga wasn't exciting for her, running hurt her ankles, and there were no good bike paths near her home. The important thing about exercise, I reminded her, is to just get moving. I asked her how she felt when she danced—and her voice perked right up! She glowed when she described how music moves her soul, and how much she loves to go out dancing. Kris decided that dancing to a few songs every day would get her excited, get her moving, and be fun, to boot! At our next session, Kris told me that she wore a wrist-monitor while she danced, which told her how aerobic her activity was. She told me she had discovered that she was getting better exercise dancing than she had been getting on her walks, which weren't nearly as enjoyable for her. Exercise is important, but it's even better and more beneficial if the activity we choose is pleasurable for us.

Exercise, which is a daunting term for moving our bodies, helps you rev up to face the day and to deal with change; it even helps you chill out. Exercise is a key ingredient to a de-stressed life, and it's one of the main ways to loosen up, move stuck energy in your body, and sweat out excess toxins. Walking around your office building or house for 20 minutes a day can increase your circulation, relax your muscles, and wake you up. Thirty minutes of speed walking, bicycling, or aerobics can work off excess stress and tension in your body and mind. Here are some important tips for getting into the exercise groove.

- Choose your exercise depending on the effect you need. For example, yoga is great for calming the mind and stretching the muscles, while running is great for revving up your energy and relieving excess stress, and playing catch with a friend is a fantastic way to connect and just have fun.

- More-challenging exercises are great for relieving anxiety and stress levels, so try more complicated activities when you're suffering from serious brain drain and body stress: Circuit training where you alternate weights and cardiovascular work, mountain biking, kickboxing, and African dance classes are all high-energy activities that will jump-start your detox. Mix it up! Your body becomes very efficient with the same movements, so alternating activities keeps both your mind and your body fresh. The more types of exercise you choose, the more muscles you will use.

## BREATHING EASY: RELEASING TOXINS THROUGH OUR BREATH AND SKIN

Coughing, sneezing, and breathing are the first ways our bodies try to remove toxins and foreign matter. As a way to deal with stress, nothing beats deep, meditative breathing. Use this technique during times of stress, before meals to bring awareness to your meal, or at the beginning of your day to focus positive intention on the work before you. I often use this technique before speaking engagements to calm and center my mind and body:

**MEDITATIVE BREATHING.** Sit straight up in a chair with your feet comfortably on the floor and your hands in your lap, resting on your thighs. Close your eyes and just be aware of your breath. Are

## Herbal Steam Bath for Lung Congestion, Asthma, Bronchitis, and Sinusitis

The following steam bath is helpful for opening air passages and soothing symptoms of respiratory problems.

**1.** Boil 4 cups of filtered water. Pour into a large heat-resistant bowl, preferably glass, ceramic, or stainless steel.

**2.** Lightly crush or chop 2 tablespoons each of fresh rosemary, thyme, and lavender and add to the hot water.

**3.** Drape a towel over your head; the towel should be large enough to form a tent over the bowl.

**4.** Holding your head about 1 foot above the steaming water, breathe the herbed vapors deeply in through your mouth and/or nose for 5 to 10 minutes. Be careful not to scald or burn your skin.

**5.** Repeat after 2 hours for further relief.

you breathing mostly from your chest in short, shallow breaths? Begin to deepen your breath by slowly inflating your belly and chest. Hold each breath on the inhale, and then exhale for a second, and slowly begin again. Do this 10 times.

**SAUNA/SWEATING.** Sweating is great for detoxification: Our pores are designed to traffic toxins out of our bodies, and the skin is the body's largest eliminating organ. Besides regular exercise, saunas and steam rooms are helpful to sweat out toxins and improve tissue functions. On a recent trip to Finland, I learned that there are two million saunas for the five million people living in this cold Nordic country. Business is often conducted in these "sweat baths," and traditionally women in Finland gave birth in them, due to their sterile cleanliness. As your metabolism and pulse rate increase due to the heat, your pores open and release sweat, your blood vessels and muscles become more flexible, and your circulation increases. Many people experience relief from colds, muscle aches, and skin problems after saunas. Feeling very alive and alert after a sauna is common. Saunas are also quite relaxing: Depression and anxiety symptoms are often relieved from these dry baths. It makes sense—when your body is relaxed and energized, your mind and emotions will be calm as well. Remember the following tips for sauna use.

- Before using a sauna, consult your physician if you are pregnant or have heart problems.

- Don't drink alcohol, eat, or use tranquilizers, stimulants, or other prescription drugs.

- Start gradually—stay in the sauna only as long as you feel comfortable on your first several visits. You may increase your time gradually with each visit.

- Be sure to drink a glass of water before and after a sauna to rehydrate your body.

- If you feel dizzy, have trouble breathing, or feel ill, leave the sauna right away.

## OTHER THERAPIES TO AID YOUR DETOX

**ENEMAS/COLONICS.** Constipation and diarrhea are common complaints from people who eat the Standard American Diet, or SAD. Constipation is usually caused by a low-fiber diet and insufficient water consumption, which cause fecal matter to become condensed and compressed in the intestines and colon. The longer your body is exposed to decaying food trapped in your intestines, the greater the risk of developing illness and disease. While a diet high in fiber will help to increase bowel movements, many people will experience great relief from enemas and colon cleansing. Different methods of colon cleansing include colon hydrotherapy, enemas, herbal supplements, and oxygen colon cleansers. Find a licensed colon therapist or try using a home kit, which can be found in many pharmacies or on the Web.

**HOT SKIN SCRUB.** Wet a washcloth or shower cloth with hot water under the faucet. Use the cloth to lightly scrub your skin all over your body to open the pores and loosen skin tissue. Performed before bed or upon waking, this quick ritual can become a wonderful tool for self-care and nurturing that helps the skin to open up and detoxify. When they perform this ritual regularly, many people report smoother, clearer skin and better circulation. Use the towel to focus your awareness on areas of concern. Do you have a sore back?

Use the towel to rub warm, soft energy into the area. Not only does the heat increase bloodflow to the area, but the simple massaging of the skin and tissue will relieve tension and relax muscles.

**SEA AND EPSOM SALT BATHS.** These bath salts are made from magnesium sulfate, a pure mineral that benefits your skin and body. Soaking in a warm tub and lightly scrubbing with added salts can soften skin and exfoliate rough patches. Soaking also provides relief from the swelling and inflammation of body aches and pains. Sea salt helps draw impurities from the skin and can diminish and calm acne, psoriasis, eczema, and rashes. The high mineral content of these salts conditions skin, leaving it feeling soft and clean. Calming and relaxing, warm baths can ease muscle tension and bring a sense of deep peacefulness.

**MASSAGE.** Used in many traditional cultures to relieve muscle tension, calm the body and mind, and move stuck energy, or "chi," massage assists the efforts of people working to detoxify their bodies. When muscles are manually manipulated with proper pressure and understanding, tissues release stuck fluids, toxins, and stress. Be sure to drink plenty of water after a massage to flush your system of freed toxins and fluids. Many books are available to instruct you on easy self-massage techniques, and there are books for couples who want to enjoy helping each other. Licensed massage schools often have discounted massage packages available for clients willing to hire a student. Rolfing, Swedish massage, deep tissue massage, and acupressure are all forms of healing massage.

# EMPTY YOUR MIND OF STRESS

A strong mind will help you see the bigger picture when you have to face the various and inevitable stresses of life. Here are some ways to integrate stress management into your daily life.

**MEDITATE.** Allow yourself a few moments of quiet time in your day. Find a secluded area in your home or office (even a bathroom stall works in a pinch!) and sit quietly with your eyes closed. Focus on drawing your breath slowly and completely in and out of your lungs. Place both hands on your belly so that you can feel the gentle rising and falling of your breath. Feel your lungs filling and emptying of air, and continue to focus on your breath for a few moments. Remember, breathing is the most important thing in life—we can all last a few days without water, and maybe a few weeks without food, but we would last only a few minutes without air! Try to enjoy a moment of silence in your mind.

**TAKE RESPONSIBILITY FOR YOUR STRESS.** The ways you react to what is happening around you—and to you—are actually in your control. Take time to assess stressful situations with care and mindfulness. Examine the many ways you can choose to respond to stress, and exercise your right to do things differently than you have in your past. Your goal should be to allow yourself to react to stress in ways that are most beneficial to you, to allow yourself, always, to do what is best for you.

**BUILD YOUR RELATIONSHIPS.** A strong support system can be the best way to ensure the success of your dreams, whether they include succeeding in detoxing your diet or taking the risks to find your life's true purpose. Cultivate strong, supportive, positive friendships. Toxic people can be a huge obstacle to getting healthy. Much research has been devoted to understanding the relationship between bodily health and healthy relationships, and the verdict is in: Positive, loving relationships create an atmosphere where self-love and healthy habits are more likely to flourish. An unhappy marriage often results in unhealthy habits; when we don't feel love in our homes, we internalize this disharmony by eating poorly and treating our bodies—and our souls— poorly.

**CREATE SHORT-TERM GOALS.** Check in with yourself and write down your short-term goals. These ideas and hopes keep us moving forward, mark our progress, and keep life manageable. Use a journal to write about your goals and how you can actually execute plans that will fulfill them. Creating plans can make goals much easier to achieve!

**ESTABLISH LONG-TERM GOALS.** Choosing your own future gives you a clean path to focus on, a purpose in life, and the strength to say no to those draining people and projects that pop up in life.

**BECOME DISCIPLINED.** Watching the Olympics, we witness the culmination of thousands of hours of hard work and practice. We marvel at the swimmer who reaches the wall first, but we don't know that she has practiced that same race 10,000 times! Don't give up! Keep moving forward toward your goals, and be kind to yourself while you find your way. Remember, you are the only one who can get you there!

**VISUALIZE THE OUTCOME.** Focus on the positive possible outcomes of this detox. Humans have a tendency to dwell on the negative, which doesn't encourage us to move forward. Imagine instead the best possible results. Get excited and creative! What do you want? How can you get that? What do you need to do to make it happen? What's standing in your way? NOTHING! The truth is, very little is usually keeping us from reaching our goals if we can train our minds to stay on a positive track. Imagining positive, creative solutions to problems and positive, rich results for our efforts will steer us away from toxic thinking and in the direction of achievement and success.

## STRESS LESSEN
### Two Simple, Powerful Tools for Reducing Stress

Since stress contributes to illness, learning to reduce stress in the body can be healing. Consider trying one of these tried-and-true methods for deeper detoxification.

**YOGA.** The positions, stretching, concentrated breathing, and meditative pace of yoga have demonstrated powerful effectiveness in relieving stress in more than 1,000 studies. And you don't even need to leave the house! DVD/VHS recordings are available covering beginning to advanced yoga techniques. All you need is a quiet, comfortable place and a desire to feel better.

**LAUGHTER.** Smiling and giggling at a problem, a situation, or ourselves is a fantastic way to feel in control and lighthearted. Keep in touch with your silly side. Being playful, silly, goofy, and able to make fun of yourself can detox almost any stressful situation. To lift a dreary mood, get to the library or video store and check out a funny movie—sometimes all we need is a little contact with a clown to make our stress melt away.

## MENTAL DETOX
### The Mind-Body Connection

Once your diet is detoxified and your body has new, cleaner fuel to run on, how can you go even deeper to cleanse your body and mind?

Mind-body medicine is a new idea in Western cultures, but practitioners of Traditional Chinese Medicine, yoga teachers, and Ayurvedic doctors from India have been treating the mind as well as the body to release people from pain and illness for centuries. Numerous studies have linked feelings of security, a strong link to community, solid coping skills, a high level of hope, and an attitude of optimism with a stronger immune system. Negative emotions such as stress, anger, depression, and hopelessness have been shown to decrease the body's ability to deal with disease and can even interfere with healing.

**Exercise:** Make a strong effort to turn your mind away from distressing emotions such as stress and anger. When these feelings come over you, begin to shift your attention to your body to calm down. Focus positive energy on your heart, gut, and head. These three areas physically manifest the stress that we feel in our minds, and sending calming energy to them can help ease the negative effects of stress. Visualize a calming pink glow settling over your heart, intestines, and forehead. Ask your heart, gut, and brain: "Why am I so upset? What is the best way to deal with this stress? How can I best protect myself and my health?" If you listen closely, you will hear the answers.

**PART THREE**

# RECIPES AND RESOURCES

# Recipes

**So now the secret is out:** This book isn't about dieting. It's about the incredible nutritional, healing powers of whole foods; how we heal ourselves by eliminating toxic, overly processed foods from our diets; and how by detoxing we begin to engage in true self-care.

Before you turn to the delicious, healthful recipes, I want to point out that I've decided against adding serving sizes. Most diet programs are built on how much protein, carbohydrate, and fat you should have in your daily diet. These generalized recommendations are, I believe, a necessary response to teasing a healthful diet out of a world that is drowning in unhealthy, overly processed foods. Now that you've made a commitment to eat whole, natural foods, you free yourself from depending on such measures. (Think about it: there are no complicated ingredient lists for fresh vegetables and fruits, whole grains, or organically raised meats.) I believe it is impossible to eat too many fresh vegetables, so attaching a serving size might inadvertently discourage you from eating what you want and what you need.

But if visualizing a serving size is helpful to you, here's my advice: I once heard that ancient monks would eat only what they could hold within their own two hands. Isn't that a beautiful thought? Your two hands make two perfect bowls. If you eat only what you can fit into both hands at each meal, I believe you will find yourself satisfied and happy.

I've also created the recipes with the idea of leftovers in mind. I've learned that having fresh, prepared foods on hand is the best way to stay on a healthy eating plan and to stay on track with your detox. To the single folks, don't be nervous about preparing full recipes. You'll soon learn the joys of having a refrigerator stocked with delicious, prepared healthy food. It reinforces the fact that you are taking good care of yourself on many levels.

## Apple Granola Muffins

*Wheat-, sugar-, and dairy-free*

| | |
|---|---|
| 1½ | cups unbleached spelt flour |
| ½ | cup whole spelt flour |
| 2 | teaspoons baking powder |
| 1 | teaspoon cinnamon |
| ½ | teaspoon sea salt |
| 1½ | cups vanilla or plain soy milk or apple juice |
| ½ | cup date sugar |
| ¼ | cup melted coconut or extra-virgin olive oil |
| 1 | teaspoon vanilla |
| 1 | medium apple, chopped |
| ½ | cup walnuts, coarsely chopped |
| 2 | tablespoons quick oats |

1. Preheat oven to 350°F. Grease a 12-cup muffin pan with melted coconut or extra-virgin olive oil. Set aside.

2. Sift the unbleached and whole spelt flours, baking powder, cinnamon, and salt together in a large mixing bowl. Stir to mix well.

3. In a medium mixing bowl, whisk together the soy milk or apple juice, sugar, oil, and vanilla.

4. Make a well in the center of the dry ingredients and pour the wet ingredients into it. Use a large spoon or rubber spatula to combine the ingredients. Stir and fold rather than beating; do not overmix. The batter should be lumpy, not smooth.

5. Carefully fold in the apples and walnuts.

6. Spoon the batter into the muffin tin, filling each cup about two-thirds full.

7. Sprinkle the oats on top of the muffins.

8. Bake for 20 to 30 minutes, or until the muffins are nicely browned and a toothpick inserted into the center of one of them comes out clean.

9. Remove from the oven and allow the muffins to rest in the tin for 5 minutes before removing them.

**YIELD: 12 MUFFINS**

# BREAKFAST PATTIES

*These keep well when individually wrapped and frozen.*

| | |
|---|---|
| 2 | tablespoons extra-virgin olive oil |
| 2 | tablespoons brown rice or spelt flour |
| 1 | tablespoon naturally brewed soy sauce (shoyu or wheat-free tamari) |
| 1½ | cups warm vegetable stock or plain soy milk |
| 1 | cup rolled oats |
| ½ | cup chopped yellow onion |
| ½ | teaspoon dried sage |
| ½ | teaspoon dried thyme |
| 1 | cup finely chopped raw nuts |
| 1 | cup cooked brown rice or other whole grain |
| 1 | cup minced shiitake or button mushrooms |

1. Place a large skillet over medium-low heat. Add the oil, flour, and soy sauce. Whisk well to combine.

2. Whisk in vegetable stock or soy milk and cook until thickened, continuing to whisk, about 2 minutes.

3. Remove from heat and add the oats, onion, sage, thyme, nuts, rice, and mushrooms. Stir well to combine and transfer entire contents to a medium mixing bowl. Allow to set at room temperature for 10 minutes, then refrigerate until cool enough to handle, about 20 minutes.

4. Preheat oven to 350°F.

5. Line a baking sheet with parchment paper.

6. Remove the mixture from refrigerator, and scoop ¼ cup of mixture into a pattiy. Place on the lined baking sheet, and continue to scoop mixture into patties until done.

7. Bake for 20 minutes, and serve. If freezing, wrap each patty individually in plastic wrap.

**YIELD: 12 PATTIES**

# Breakfast Tofu Scramble for One

*Draining tofu releases excess water stored on the inside of the block. To press out the water, set the tofu on the bottom side of a plate, placed at a slight tilt in a kitchen sink. Add another plate to the top of the tofu and weigh it down slightly. Allow to drain for 10 minutes. This process will reduce the amount of water in the recipe. Double the recipe for two people.*

| | |
|---|---|
| 1 | tablespoon extra-virgin olive oil |
| 1/4 | cup chopped red onion |
| 1 | clove garlic, minced |
| 2 | sun-dried tomatoes, chopped (use either oil-packed or the reconstituted dry version) |
| 1 | cup fresh baby spinach leaves, washed and dried |
| 1/4 | teaspoon red pepper flakes |
| 1/4 | teaspoon turmeric powder |
| 2 | teaspoons naturally brewed soy sauce (shoyu or tamari) |
| 1 | teaspoon miso paste |
| 1 | tablespoon water |
| 1/2 | block soft tofu, rinsed and drained |
| | Corn or flour tortillas (optional) |

1. Heat a medium skillet over medium heat. Add the oil and sauté the onion for 1 minute.

2. Add the garlic, tomatoes, spinach, red pepper flakes, and turmeric. Stir well to combine.

3. In a small bowl, combine the soy sauce, miso paste, and water. Whisk until well combined, and pour over the vegetables.

4. Crumble the tofu with your fingers into small, bite-size bits. Add the tofu to the skillet and stir well to combine the tofu with the vegetables. Cook for 1 minute. Serve warm with the tortillas, if desired.

**YIELD: 1½ CUPS**

# Hearty Morning Oatmeal Porridge

| | |
|---|---|
| 1 | cup whole oat groats |
| 2½ | cups water |
| 1 | cup freshly squeezed orange juice |
| ¼ | teaspoon ground nutmeg |
| ¼ | teaspoon cinnamon |
| | Tiny pinch of sea salt |
| 6 | tablespoons brown rice syrup, pure maple syrup, agave nectar, or date sugar |
| 6 | tablespoons chopped nuts |

1. Place the groats, water, orange juice, nutmeg, cinnamon, and salt in a medium saucepan and stir to combine. Cover and bring to a boil.

2. Reduce heat to low and cook for 50 to 60 minutes, until the oats are soft and the liquid is gone. Remove from the heat and let sit, covered, for 2 to 5 minutes. Stir in the syrup, nectar, or sugar and top with the nuts. Serve hot.

**YIELD: 3½ CUPS**

# Orange Date Scones

*Wheat- and dairy-free.*

|   |   |
|---|---|
| 1 | cup unbleached spelt flour |
| 1/2 | cup whole spelt flour |
| 1/4 | teaspoon salt |
| 2 | teaspoons non-aluminum baking powder |
| 1/3 | cup pitted dates, cut into quarters (about 6 dates) |
| 1/3 | cup walnuts or pecans, coarsely chopped |
| 3 | tablespoons extra-virgin olive oil |
| 1/4 | cup maple or brown rice syrup |
| 2 | teaspoons fresh orange zest (zest of 1 large orange) |
| 1/3 | cup orange juice |

1. Preheat oven to 425°F.

2. Mix the unbleached spelt flour, whole spelt flour, salt, and baking powder together in a large mixing bowl. Add the dates and nuts and stir to combine. Set aside.

3. In a medium mixing bowl, combine the oil, syrup, orange zest, and orange juice. Whisk together to combine.

4. Pour the wet mixture into the dry mixture and mix with a wooden spoon until just combined (do not overmix, as this will make the scones tough).

5. Using a 1/3-cup measuring cup and a rubber spatula, scoop 6 portions of the dough onto a baking sheet lined with parchment paper.

6. Bake for 10 to 12 minutes, until scones are lightly browned at the edges.

**YIELD: 6 SCONES**

# Power Morning Shake

*This is one of Morgan's and my favorite breakfasts—quick, filling, delicious, and full of nutrients!*

| | |
|---|---|
| 1 | banana, frozen or fresh |
| 1 | cup berries, frozen or fresh |
| 1/4 | cup raw nuts* or 1 scoop of protein powder |
| 2 | cups water, fresh juice, or soy, rice, or almond milk |
| 1 | teaspoon vitamin C powder |
| 1 | tablespoon chlorophyll-rich powder (chlorella, spirulina, etc.) |
| 2 | tablespoons aloe vera juice |
| 1 | tablespoon ground flaxseeds or flaxseed oil |
| 1/2 | cup yogurt (optional) |

1. Combine the banana, berries, nuts or protein powder, water or juice or milk, vitamin C powder, chlorophyll-rich powder, aloe vera juice, flaxseeds or oil, and yogurt (if using) in a blender. Blend until smooth. Serve immediately.

**YIELD: 4 CUPS**

***Note:*** *Just 1/4 cup of walnuts gives you a day's worth of omega-3 fatty acids. If you are allergic to walnuts, use an additional tablespoon of ground flaxseeds, which offer 670 milligrams of omega-3 per tablespoon.*

# Wheat-Free Pancakes with Blueberry Syrup

| | |
|---|---|
| 1 | cup blueberries, fresh or thawed frozen |
| 1 | cup brown rice syrup |
| 1 | cup buckwheat flour |
| 1 | cup corn flour |
| 2 | teaspoons baking powder |
| 1 | teaspoon vanilla extract |
| | Pinch of sea salt |
| 1½ | cups almond milk or soy milk |
| 1 | tablespoon orange zest |
| 1 | cup applesauce |
| 3 | tablespoons water |
| | Unrefined organic coconut oil, olive oil, or unrefined, organic canola oil for skillet |

1. Combine the blueberries and brown rice syrup in a small saucepan over low heat. Cook for 3 minutes, bringing the syrup to a low simmer. Turn off the heat and set aside.

2. In a large mixing bowl, sift together the buckwheat flour, corn flour, and baking powder.

3. In a medium bowl, combine the vanilla, salt, milk, orange zest, applesauce, and water.

4. Pour the wet ingredients into the dry, and mix lightly. Do not overmix, as it will cause the pancakes to be tough.

5. Heat a large skillet over medium-high, and add 1 tablespoon of desired oil. Tilt the skillet to coat the bottom of the pan with oil.

6. Pour ¼-cup portions of pancake mix onto the hot skillet and cook for 2 minutes, until lightly browned and bubbles form. Flip the pancakes and cook for 1 additional minute.

7. Repeat process until all the batter is gone, re-oiling the skillet between batches.

8. Top with blueberry syrup.

**YIELD: 15 4" PANCAKES**

# ALMOND MILK

*A delicious and easy dairy-free milk substitute.*

| | |
|---|---|
| 2 | cups unsalted slivered almonds |
| 4 | cups water |
| 1 | teaspoon pure vanilla extract |
| 2-4 | tablespoons maple syrup (to taste) |

1. Combine the almonds and 2 cups of the water in a blender.

2. Pulse for 20 seconds and then blend on a low setting for 2 minutes. With the blender still running, add the rest of the water a little at a time, then the vanilla and maple syrup.

3. Blend for 1 minute more. Line a colander with a cheesecloth and pour the milk through it. Squeeze the excess out of the almond meat in the cloth.

**YIELD: 3½ CUPS**

# SWEET AND SPICY CHAI TEA

*A traditional Indian beverage with a kick!*

| | |
|---|---|
| 2 | whole cardamom pods |
| 1 | piece (1") cinnamon stick |
| 3 | whole black peppercorns |
| 1 | piece (½") fresh ginger |
| 1 | tablespoon brown rice syrup or maple syrup |
| 2 | cups soy, rice, or fresh nut milk |

1. Combine the cardamom, cinnamon, peppercorns, ginger, syrup, and milk in a small pot and place over medium heat. Cover and bring the mixture to a low simmer. Lower the heat to low and cook, uncovered, for 4 minutes.

2. Serve hot.

**YIELD: 2 CUPS**

# Safely Sweet Lemonade

*Stevia extract can be found in either liquid or powder form in the "dietary supplements" aisle of health food stores. It is a remarkable aid for people with diabetes and blood sugar concerns, as it does not affect blood sugar levels or exacerbate yeast conditions.*

| | |
|---|---|
| 8 | cups filtered water |
| ½ | cup fresh lemon juice |
| ½–1 | teaspoon liquid stevia extract |

1. Combine the water, lemon juice, and stevia in a large glass pitcher and serve over ice for a refreshing beverage.

**YIELD: 8½ CUPS**


# Sunny Citrus Tea

| | |
|---|---|
| 6 | cups filtered water, divided |
| 2 | herbal tea bags |
| 2 | tablespoons maple syrup or brown rice syrup |
| 1 | whole clove |
| 1 | piece (½″) cinnamon stick |
| 2 | cups freshly squeezed orange juice |
| 2 | tablespoons lemon juice |

1. Bring 2 cups of the water to a boil in a small saucepan. Add the tea bags, syrup, clove, and cinnamon stick. Cover, remove from heat, and allow to steep for 5 minutes.

2. Remove the tea bags, clove, and cinnamon stick and allow the mixture to cool for 15 minutes.

3. Stir in the remaining 4 cups water and the orange and lemon juices.

4. Serve cold over ice.

**YIELD: 8 CUPS**

# Cold and Flu Tea

| 4 | cups water |
|---|---|
| 3 | slices fresh ginger—*warming, immune enhancer, relieves nausea and headache* |
| 6 | fresh sage leaves—*nervous system stimulation, helpful for throat conditions* |
| 2 to 3 | fresh thyme sprigs—*antibiotic, antiviral* |
| | Fresh juice from $1/2$ lemon—*vitamin C, antibacterial* |
| 1 | piece ($1/2$") cinnamon stick—*warming, digestive support* |

1. In a pot, bring the water to a boil. Remove from the heat and add the ginger, sage, thyme, lemon juice, and cinnamon.

2. Steep for 5 to 15 minutes. Strain and drink twice a day.

**YIELD: 4 CUPS**

# Liver Tonic Tea

| 4 | cups water |
|---|---|
| 4 | slices fresh ginger, cut to thickness of a quarter—*warming, immune enhancer* |
| 1 | tablespoon dried or fresh chamomile—*sweet flavor, calming* |
| 2 | slices ($1/2$" each) burdock root—*liver support, blood cleanser* |
| 1 | piece (1") dried dandelion root—*liver support* |
| 2 | teaspoons dried or fresh mint—*sweet flavor, digestive support* |

1. In a pot, bring the water to a boil. Remove from the heat and add the ginger, chamomile, burdock, dandelion, and mint.

2. Steep for 10 to 15 minutes. Strain and drink once a day.

**YIELD: 4 CUPS**

# BEDTIME RELAX TEA

    4    cups water

    1    teaspoon dried or fresh chamomile—*sweet, calming*

    1    teaspoon dried lavender—*stress and depression relief*

    1    teaspoon dried mint—*sweet, digestive aid*

    1    teaspoon fennel seeds—*supports kidneys, liver, and lungs*

    1    teaspoon dried lemon balm—*calming, aromatic*

1. In a pot, bring the water to a boil. Remove from the heat and add the chamomile, lavender, mint, fennel, and lemon balm.

2. Steep for 5 to 15 minutes. Strain and drink once a day.

**YIELD: 4 CUPS**

# Warming Winter Digestive Tea

| 4 | cups water |
|---|---|
| 3 | slices fresh ginger, cut to thickness of a quarter—*warming, immune enhancer* |
| 1 | piece (1") licorice root—*antiviral, antibacterial, fights depression* |
| 1 | piece (¹⁄₂") cinnamon stick—*warming, digestive support, useful for diabetes* |
| 1 | tablespoon organic orange rind—*sweet* |
| 1 | tablespoon dried parsley—*digestive aid* |
| 1 | teaspoon dried lemon balm—*relaxing, aromatic* |
| 1 | clove—*warming, digestive aid* |

1. In a pot, bring the water to a boil. Remove from the heat and add the ginger, licorice root, cinnamon stick, orange rind, parsley, lemon balm, and clove.

2. Steep for 5 to 15 minutes. Strain and drink twice a day.

**4 CUPS**

# Watermelon Cooler

| 8 | cups watermelon, deseeded and chopped |
|---|---|
| ¹⁄₄ | teaspoon liquid stevia extract |
| 2 | tablespoons lime juice |
| 2 | cups ice cubes |
| | Fresh mint leaves |

1. Combine the watermelon, stevia, and lime juice in a blender and puree until smooth. Add the ice and process until the ice is finely crushed.

2. Divide mixture among pretty glasses, garnish with mint leaves, and serve immediately.

**YIELD: 10 CUPS**

# Corn, Mushroom, and Potato Chowder

3     tablespoons extra-virgin olive oil, divided

2     cups chopped yellow onions

6     cups vegetable stock, divided

3     cups cubed potatoes, peeled and cut into 1" cubes

1     teaspoon sea salt

$\frac{1}{2}$     teaspoon freshly ground black pepper

4     ears corn, kernels scraped off into a bowl, or one 10-ounce package thawed frozen corn

1     cup thinly sliced mushrooms (button, shiitake, or chanterelle)

     Fresh parsley

1. Heat a 6 to 8 quart pot over medium heat. Add 2 tablespoons of the oil and sauté the onions for about 5 minutes, stirring often.

2. Add 3 cups of the vegetable stock and the potatoes, salt, and pepper. Cover and bring to a boil, reduce heat to a simmer, and cook for 10 minutes, or until the potatoes are tender.

3. Add the corn and remaining stock to the pot and cook for another 5 minutes.

4. While the corn cooks, heat a medium skillet over medium heat and add the remaining 1 tablespoon of oil. Sauté the mushrooms for 5 minutes, stirring often. Add to the soup and stir.

5. Garnish with parsley and serve hot.

**YIELD: 8 CUPS**

# "Creamy" Carrot Soup

1 tablespoon extra-virgin olive oil

1 cup chopped yellow onion

2 cloves garlic, minced

2 teaspoons sea salt

1 teaspoon fennel seeds

4 cups carrots, scrubbed, dried, and cut into 1" coin slices

4 cups unsalted vegetable stock or filtered water

Fresh dill or parsley

1. Heat a 4 quart pot over medium heat and add the oil.

2. Add the onion and garlic with the salt, stir to coat the vegetables with oil, and sauté for 3 to 4 minutes.

3. Add the fennel seeds, carrots, and stock or water, cover, and bring to a boil over high heat.

4. Reduce heat to a low simmer and cook until carrots are tender, about 20 minutes.

5. Blend soup in the pot with a stick/immersion blender, or transfer to a blender 1 cup at a time and blend until smooth.

6. Garnish with the dill or parsley.

**YIELD: 5 CUPS**

# "Creamy" Potato Leek Soup

| | |
|---|---|
| 1 | tablespoon extra-virgin olive oil |
| 2 | leeks, white and light green parts washed and sliced into $1/4''$ slices |
| 2 | cups chopped yellow onion |
| $1/2$ | teaspoon sea salt |
| 3 | cloves garlic, minced |
| 2 | large Yukon Gold potatoes (about 1 pound), peeled and cubed into $1/2''$ cubes |
| 4 | cups vegetable stock |
| 2–3 | teaspoons fresh rosemary leaves |

1. Heat a 4 quart pot over medium heat and add the oil.

2. Add the leeks, onion, and sea salt and sauté for about 5 minutes, stirring often, until the onion begins to turn translucent.

3. Add the garlic and stir well. Cook for 1 minute more.

4. Add the potatoes and vegetable stock, cover, and bring to a boil. Reduce heat to simmer. Cook for 20 minutes.

5. Remove the soup from heat and use an immersion/stick blender to blend the soup in the pot or ladle the soup into a blender, 1 cup at a time. Blend the soup with the fresh rosemary leaves until smooth and free of chunks. Pour smooth soup into a heat-proof bowl and continue until all of the soup has been blended.

6. Transfer the blended soup back to the original soup pot and warm over low heat until heated through. Serve hot.

**YIELD: 7 CUPS**

# Milanese Tomato Soup

| | |
|---|---|
| 1 | tablespoon extra-virgin olive oil |
| 1 | cup chopped yellow onion |
| 2 | cloves garlic, minced |
| 1/3 | cup chopped celery |
| 4 | cups vegetable stock |
| 1 | 28-ounce can crushed tomatoes, with liquid |
| 1/2 | cup shredded carrot |
| 1/4 | cup tomato paste |
| 1 | tablespoon maple or brown rice syrup |
| 1 | teaspoon sea salt |
| 1/2 | teaspoon freshly ground black pepper |
| 2 | cups trimmed and chopped spinach |
| 1/2 | cup chopped fresh basil |
| | Fresh Italian (flat-leaf) parsley |

1. Set a 6 to 8 quart pot over medium heat and add the oil and onion. Sauté for 5 minutes.

2. Add the garlic and celery; stir well, and sauté for 1 more minute.

3. Add the vegetable stock, tomatoes, carrot, tomato paste, syrup, sea salt, and pepper. Stir well, cover and bring to a boil.

4. Add the spinach and basil, cover, and remove from heat. Keep covered for 5 minutes before serving. Serve hot, garnishing each bowl with parsley.

**YIELD: 8 CUPS**

# Tomato Vegetable Soup

*Add 1 cup of cooked beans or leftover cubed protein for added protein.*

| | |
|---|---|
| 1 | tablespoon extra-virgin olive oil |
| ½ | cup chopped red onion |
| ¼ | teaspoon sea salt |
| 2 | cloves garlic, minced |
| ½ | cup shredded carrot |
| ½ | cup chopped celery |
| 1 | 24-ounce can diced tomatoes |
| 3 | cups vegetable stock |
| ¼ | teaspoon freshly ground black pepper |
| | Fresh parsley leaves |

1. Heat a 4 quart pot over medium heat and add the oil.

2. Add the onion and salt and sauté for 2 minutes. Add the garlic and sauté for 1 minute more.

3. Add the carrot, celery, tomatoes, stock, and pepper and set over medium-low heat. Stir a few times and cover. Bring to a low simmer and cook for 20 minutes, stirring occasionally.

4. Garnish with parsley leaves and serve hot.

**YIELD: 7 CUPS**

# Miso Stew

*Gourmet* magazine said this stew was *"as healthy as it gets!"*

| | |
|---|---|
| $\frac{1}{3}$ | cup rinsed and drained quinoa |
| $4\frac{1}{2}$ | cups filtered water |
| 1 | piece (1") kombu seaweed |
| 2 | tablespoons arame seaweed |
| 2 | teaspoons extra-virgin olive oil |
| $\frac{1}{2}$ | cup chopped yellow onion |
| 2 | cloves garlic, thinly sliced |
| $\frac{1}{2}$ | cup chopped firm tofu, rinsed and drained |
| $\frac{1}{2}$ | cup sliced carrot |
| 3 | fresh shiitake mushrooms, sliced |
| 1-2 | tablespoons miso paste |
| 1 | cup thinly sliced bok choy or napa cabbage |
| 1 | teaspoon naturally brewed soy sauce (shoyu or tamari) |
| 2 | tablespoons sliced scallions |
| $\frac{1}{2}$ | teaspoon dulse flakes |

1. Combine the quinoa with 1 cup of the filtered water and the kombu in a small saucepan. Cover, set over medium-high heat, and bring to a boil. Reduce to low and simmer for 20 minutes, or until the quinoa is cooked through.

2. Meanwhile, soak the arame in 1 cup of filtered water. Set aside.

3. In a medium saucepan, heat the oil over medium heat, add the onion, and sauté for 5 minutes, until it begins to brown. Add the garlic and continue to sauté for 30 seconds, stirring a couple of times.

4. Add the tofu and the remaining 2½ cups filtered water, carrot, and mushrooms. Cover and simmer on medium-low heat for 5 minutes. Remove from heat.

5. Remove the kombu from the quinoa and discard it. Add the quinoa to the stew. Stir to combine.

6. Measure the miso into a small bowl and add ½ cup of the hot stew liquid from the pot to the bowl. Using a whisk, dissolve the miso into the liquid and return the mixture to the saucepan. Do not boil or simmer the miso, as this destroys the beneficial microorganisms.

7. Add the bok choy or napa cabbage and the soy sauce to the pot, and stir to combine. This will wilt the greens just a bit.

8. Rinse and drain the arame and add to the stew.

9. Measure stew into two bowls and garnish with the scallions and a sprinkle of dulse flakes.

**YIELD: 4½ CUPS**

# Neptune's Noodle Soup

$\frac{1}{2}$ block extra-firm tofu, cut into 1" cubes, drained, and rinsed

2 tablespoons extra-virgin olive oil, divided

5 teaspoons naturally brewed soy sauce (shoyu or wheat-free tamari), divided

1 teaspoon garlic powder

1 teaspoon onion powder

1 cup pasta shells, uncooked

1 cup sliced yellow onion

5 cloves garlic, minced

$\frac{1}{2}$ cup sliced carrot

$\frac{1}{2}$ cup sliced celery

$\frac{1}{2}$ teaspoon ground red pepper

6 cups unsalted vegetable stock

1 sheet nori, cut into 1" strips

2 tablespoons dulse flakes

1. Preheat oven to 400°F.

2. Combine the tofu, 1 tablespoon of the oil, 3 teaspoons of the soy sauce, the garlic powder, and onion powder in a small mixing bowl and toss to coat.

3. Spread the tofu cubes and the marinade evenly in a glass casserole dish and bake for 20 minutes, stirring every 5 minutes. Remove from oven and set aside.

4. While the tofu is cooking, cook the pasta according to the directions on the package. Drain and rinse under cool water to stop the cooking. Set aside.

5. Set a 6 to 8 quart pot over medium heat and add the remaining 1 tablespoon oil. Add the onion and sauté until it begins to turn brown and caramelize, about 10 minutes.

6. Add the garlic, carrot, celery, pepper, and the remaining 2 teaspoons of soy sauce and sauté until tender, about 5 minutes.

7. Pour in the stock, and add the nori and dulse flakes. Turn the heat to high, cover, and bring to a boil.

8. Turn off the heat, uncover, and add the cooked pasta and tofu.

**YIELD: 10 CUPS**

# Vietnamese Noodle Soup

|       |                                                      |
|-------|------------------------------------------------------|
| 8     | cups water                                           |
| 1     | piece (2") kombu                                     |
| 8     | shiitake mushrooms, thinly sliced                    |
| 2     | whole cloves                                         |
| 1/2   | cup thinly sliced yellow onion                       |
| 1     | piece (1") ginger, peeled and sliced thinly into matchsticks |
| 1     | cup shredded carrot                                  |
| 1     | cup sliced napa cabbage                              |
| 2     | teaspoons red pepper flakes                          |
| 1/2   | cup sliced green onions, both green and white parts  |
| 1/4   | cup naturally brewed soy sauce (shoyu or wheat-free tamari) |
| 1 1/2 | cups (15-ounce can) white beans, drained             |
| 1/4   | pound (about 2 cups) dry rice or mung bean noodles   |
| 1/4   | cup fresh basil                                      |
| 1/4   | cup fresh cilantro leaves                            |
| 6     | lime wedges                                          |

1. Combine the water, kombu, mushrooms, and cloves in a 6 to 8 quart pot and place over high heat, cover, and bring to a boil.

2. Remove the cloves, and add the onion, ginger, carrot, cabbage, red pepper flakes, green onions, soy sauce, and beans to the broth. Bring soup back to a simmer and cook for 5 minutes, stirring occasionally.

3. Add the noodles and stir. Remove the pot from the heat, cover, and allow to sit for 5 minutes.

4. Serve the soup in individual bowls topped with the basil, cilantro, and a wedge of lime.

**YIELD: 12 CUPS**

## CHICKPEA LEMON SPINACH SALAD

| | |
|---|---|
| 3 | cups cooked or 2 15-ounce cans chickpeas. rinsed and drained |
| 1 | cup finely chopped parsley or baby spinach leaves |
| ¼ | cup extra-virgin olive oil |
| ¼ | cup freshly squeezed lemon juice (about 2 lemons) |
| ½-1 | teaspoon sea salt |
| ½ | teaspoon freshly ground black pepper |

1. Put the chickpeas into a large mixing bowl.

2. Add the parsley or spinach, oil, lemon juice, salt, and pepper, and stir well with a wooden spoon to combine.

3. Allow the flavors to marry by marinating in the refrigerator for at least an hour.

4. Remove from the refrigerator and stir well before serving. Serve cold or at room temperature.

**YIELD: 3 CUPS**

# Herbed Garden Salad

| | |
|---|---|
| 3 | cups tomatoes, seeded and chopped |
| 1 | avocado, pitted, peeled, and chopped into 1/2" cubes |
| 1/4 | cup chopped white onion |
| 1/4 | cup chopped red bell pepper |
| 1/4 | cup chopped orange bell pepper |
| 1/4 | cup chopped fresh Italian (flat-leaf) parsley |
| 1/4 | cup thinly sliced fresh basil leaves |
| 2 | tablespoons thinly sliced fresh chives |
| 2 | tablespoons thinly sliced fresh tarragon |
| 2 | tablespoons thinly sliced fresh dill |
| 4 | tablespoons extra-virgin olive oil |
| 3 | tablespoons lemon juice |
| 1 | teaspoon sea salt |
| | Fresh black pepper to taste |

1. In a large mixing bowl, combine the tomatoes, avocado, onion, red and orange bell peppers, parsley, basil, chives, tarragon, and dill.
2. In a small mixing bowl, whisk the oil, lemon juice, salt, and pepper. Pour over the herbed mix and stir well to coat the vegetables.

**YIELD: 4 CUPS**

# HERBED QUINOA SALAD

  2    cups filtered water

  1    cup quinoa, rinsed and drained three times

  1    teaspoon sea salt, divided

  3    tablespoons extra-virgin olive oil

  1    clove garlic, minced

  2    tablespoons finely chopped Italian (flat-leaf)
       parsley

  ½    teaspoon finely chopped fresh rosemary

  ½    teaspoon finely chopped fresh thyme

  ¼    teaspoon freshly ground black pepper

  2    fresh basil leaves, shredded

1. In a small pot, bring the water to a boil over high heat and add the quinoa and ½ teaspoon of the salt. Cover, lower heat to a simmer, and cook for 20 minutes, or until all of the water has evaporated.

2. Meanwhile, place a large skillet over medium-high heat and add the oil and garlic. Sauté for 20 seconds.

3. Stir in the parsley, rosemary, and thyme and season with the remaining ½ teaspoon of salt and the pepper. After 30 seconds, remove the skillet from the heat and set aside.

4. When the quinoa is cooked, add it to the skillet and stir to combine. Add the basil and stir again. Serve immediately.

**YIELD: 4 CUPS**

# Refreshing and Cleansing Radish Salad

| | |
|---|---|
| 2 | cups peeled and thinly sliced daikon (Japanese white radish) |
| 1 | cup thinly sliced green apple, sliced into half-moons |
| 1/3 | cup grated carrot |
| 1/4 | cup thinly sliced red onion, sliced into half-moons |
| 1 | red radish, grated |
| 1/4 | cup freshly squeezed orange juice |
| 2 | teaspoons brown rice syrup |
| 1 | teaspoon freshly squeezed lime juice |
| 1 | teaspoon sea salt |
| 10 | leaves fresh mint and cilantro (optional) |

1. Combine the daikon, apple, carrot, onion, and red radish in a large mixing bowl.

2. In a small mixing bowl, whisk together the orange juice, rice syrup, lime juice, and sea salt.

3. Pour the liquid over the vegetables and toss well to combine.

4. Garnish with the mint and cilantro.

**YIELD: 3 CUPS**

# Roasted Veggies and Savory Quinoa Salad

        2    cups scrubbed beets, cut into 1/2" cubes

        1    cup scrubbed carrots, cut into 1" cubes

        1    cup yellow onion, cut into 1" cubes

        1    cup scrubbed parsnip, cut into 1" cubes

        2    tablespoons extra-virgin olive oil

      1–2    teaspoons fresh rosemary

     1 1/2    teaspoons sea salt

        2    cups vegetable stock

        1    cup quinoa, rinsed and drained

1. Preheat oven to 350°F.

2. Combine the beets, carrots, onion, and parsnip in a large mixing bowl and toss with the oil, rosemary, and salt.

3. Lay out the vegetables evenly on a baking sheet. Bake for 30 to 40 minutes, stirring once or twice during roasting, until the vegetables are tender and beginning to brown.

4. Meanwhile, bring the stock to a boil in a 4 quart pot, add the quinoa, cover, and lower heat to a simmer. Cook for 20 minutes, or until the liquid is cooked off. Remove from the heat and set aside.

5. When veggies and quinoa are finished, toss them together and serve.

**YIELD: 5 CUPS**

# Walnut Lentil Salad

$1\frac{1}{2}$    cups cooked brown lentils, cooled and drained

$\frac{1}{4}$    cup sliced green onions, green part only

1    cup packed thinly sliced baby spinach

8    sun-dried tomatoes, packed in oil, drained and chopped ($\frac{1}{4}$ cup)

$\frac{1}{4}$    cup chopped walnuts

2    tablespoons extra-virgin olive oil

1    tablespoon balsamic vinegar

1    teaspoon Dijon mustard

1    teaspoon chopped fresh rosemary

1    clove garlic, crushed

$\frac{1}{2}$    teaspoon sea salt

$\frac{1}{4}$    teaspoon freshly ground black pepper

1. In a large mixing bowl, combine the lentils, green onions, spinach, tomatoes, and walnuts. Mix well with a large wooden spoon or rubber spatula and set aside.

2. In a small mixing bowl, combine the oil, vinegar, mustard, rosemary, garlic, salt, and pepper and whisk together. Pour over the lentil salad and mix well.

3. Allow the salad to set at room temperature for at least 30 minutes, stirring a few times before serving.

**YIELD: 3 CUPS**

# Warm Potato and Kale Salad

3  large Yukon Gold or other baking potatoes (about 1¹/₂ pounds), cut into ¹/₂″ cubes

2  teaspoons sea salt, divided

2  tablespoons extra-virgin olive oil

¹/₂  cup chopped yellow onion

2  cloves garlic, sliced

4  cups kale, washed, drained, and chopped into thin strips

1  cup chopped tomatoes, seeded

1. Bring a 6 to 8 quart pot of water to a boil, and add the potatoes and 1 teaspoon salt. Cover, reduce to a simmer, and simmer for 15 minutes.

2. Meanwhile, heat a large skillet over medium heat and add the oil. Sauté the onion, stirring often, for 5 minutes. Add the garlic, stir well, and cook for 1 minute more.

3. Add the kale, tomatoes, and the remaining 1 teaspoon salt to the sautéed onions, stir well to combine, and cook for 2 minutes. Cover and remove from heat.

4. Drain the cooked potatoes and add them to the sautéed onions and kale. Stir well to combine and serve.

**YIELD: 4¹/₂ CUPS**

# Asparagus, Bok Choy, and Tofu Stir-Fry

*You may wish to serve this dish over brown rice.*

| | |
|---|---|
| 1 | tablespoon toasted sesame oil |
| 1 | clove garlic, sliced thinly |
| 1 | piece ($^1/_2$″) fresh ginger, peeled and sliced into matchsticks |
| 2 | tablespoons naturally brewed soy sauce (shoyu or tamari) |
| 10 | asparagus spears, bottom 2 inches of woody stem discarded, and remainder cut into 2″ pieces |
| 4 | cups chopped bok choy |
| $^1/_2$ | package (7 ounces) firm tofu, rinsed, drained, and cut into bite-size cubes |
| 2 | tablespoons water |

1. Heat a large skillet or wok over high heat.

2. Add the oil and sauté the garlic and ginger, stirring constantly for 30 seconds. Do not allow the garlic to burn or turn brown as it will impart a very bitter taste.

3. Add the soy sauce, asparagus, bok choy, and tofu and stir well. Add the water and allow to steam as you continue to stir often for 5 minutes. This will lightly steam the vegetables and tofu.

4. Serve hot.

**YIELD: 6$^1/_2$ CUPS**

# Baked Tempeh

> 3    8-ounce packages tempeh, sliced into
>      $\frac{1}{2}"$ × 3" slices, 8 slices for each package
>
> $\frac{1}{4}$    cup extra-virgin olive oil
>
> $\frac{1}{4}$    cup naturally brewed soy sauce (shoyu or
>      tamari) or Bragg's liquid aminos

1. Preheat oven to 375°F.

2. Place the sliced tempeh in a 13" × 9" glass baking dish. Whisk the oil and soy sauce or aminos together, and pour over the tempeh.

3. Bake for 15 minutes.

4. Remove the tempeh from the oven and allow to cool for 5 minutes. Serve warm or cold with barbeque dipping sauce.

**YIELD: 24 SLICES**

# BLACK BEAN AND SWEET POTATO CHILI

*This is delicious served over brown rice. Freeze individual portions for great leftovers!*

| | |
|---|---|
| 2 | tablespoons extra-virgin olive oil |
| 1 | medium red onion, chopped |
| 1 | red pepper, chopped |
| 4 | cloves garlic, minced |
| 2 | teaspoons sea salt |
| 1 | large sweet potato, cut into ½" cubes |
| | Zest and juice of 1 lime |
| 1 | can (28 ounces) diced tomatoes |
| 4 | cans (15 ounces each) black beans, rinsed and drained (or 6 cups freshly cooked) |
| 1 | jalapeño chile pepper, seeded and chopped |
| 1 | tablespoon cumin |
| 1 | tablespoon chili powder |
| 1 | teaspoon cocoa powder |
| 1 | lime, cut into wedges |
| 1 | cup chopped cilantro leaves, washed and dried |

1. Warm the oil in a large pan over medium heat and add the onion, red pepper, garlic, and salt. Sauté until soft, about 4 minutes.

2. Add the sweet potato and lime zest, cook 10 to 15 minutes more, continuing to stir occasionally.

3. Add the tomatoes, black beans, jalapeño, lime juice, cumin, chili powder, and cocoa, bring to a simmer, cover, and cook for 10 minutes.

4. Serve over brown rice with lime wedges and cilantro.

**YIELD: 11 CUPS**

# Corn and Kidney Bean Chili

    3   ears fresh corn, husks and silk removed

    2   tablespoons extra-virgin olive oil

    1   medium yellow onion, chopped

    2   cloves garlic, minced

    2   teaspoons sea salt

    1   tablespoon chili powder

    1   teaspoon cumin

  1/2   teaspoon ground red pepper

    1   can (15 ounces) kidney beans, rinsed and
        drained, or 1 1/2 cups fresh cooked kidney
        beans

    1   can (24 ounces) plain crushed tomatoes

1. Cut the kernels off of the cobs and set aside.

2. Set a 4 quart pot over medium heat, and add the oil and onion.

3. Sauté for 2 minutes, and add the corn, garlic, salt, chili powder, cumin, and ground red pepper. Stir well and cook for 2 minutes more.

4. Add the beans and tomatoes to the corn and onion mixture, stir well, and cover.

5. Turn the heat to low, and allow to simmer for 20 minutes.

6. Taste and add more salt, if desired.

**YIELD: 5 CUPS**

# Broccoli and Miso Calzones

*This dish combines powerful cruciferous vegetables and fermented foods in one tasty meal.*

| | |
|---|---|
| 1 | packet (2¼ teaspoons) dry yeast |
| 1 | cup warm water (105–115°F), divided |
| 1 | tablespoon maple syrup |
| 1³/₄ | cups + 2 tablespoons whole wheat or whole spelt flour |
| 1 | cup + 3 tablespoons unbleached white or spelt flour |
| 1¹/₂ | teaspoons sea salt, divided |
| 3 | cups chopped fresh broccoli florets |
| 1 | tablespoon extra-virgin olive oil |
| ¹/₂ | cup chopped yellow onion |
| ¹/₂ | cup shredded carrot |
| 6 | black olives, chopped |
| 1 | clove garlic, minced |
| 2 | tablespoons warm water |
| 2 | tablespoons miso paste |
| ¹/₄ | teaspoon freshly ground black pepper |

1. In a large mixing bowl, dissolve the yeast in ¼ cup of the water (about 105°-110°F). Let stand for 5 minutes.

2. Combine the remaining ¾ cup warm water and maple syrup; add to yeast mixture, stirring gently.

3. Gradually whisk in 1¾ cups whole wheat or whole spelt flour, the unbleached white or spelt flour, and ½ teaspoon salt to make a soft dough. Do not overmix, as this will result in a tough dough.

4. Sprinkle 1 tablespoon of whole wheat or whole spelt flour evenly over a clean, dry work surface. Turn the dough out onto the floured work surface, and knead until smooth and elastic, about 8 minutes.

5. Place the dough in a large mixing bowl that has been lightly coated with extra-virgin olive oil, and turn the dough to get a light coating of oil all over the dough. Cover dough with a clean kitchen towel and allow to rise in a warm, draft-free place for 45 minutes, or until doubled in bulk. (*Note:* Placing the rising dough on top of the refrigerator or high up somewhere will provide a perfect place for rising!)

6. Meanwhile, bring a 4 quart pot of water to a boil and add the remaining 1 teaspoon of sea salt. Quickly cook the broccoli florets in the boiling water for 1 minute. Drain, and rinse with cold water to stop the cooking process.

7. Heat a medium skillet over medium heat and add the oil. Add the onion, carrot, olives, and garlic and sauté for 2 minutes. Mix the warm water and miso together and pour over the vegetables. Turn off the heat and add the broccoli. Stir well to combine and sprinkle with pepper.

8. Preheat oven to 425°F.

9. Punch down the dough and divide into 6 equal portions. Shape each portion into a ball, cover with a clean dish towel, and allow to rest for 5 minutes.

10. Sprinkle the remaining 1 tablespoon of whole wheat or whole spelt flour over a clean work surface. Roll one portion into a 7-inch circle. Repeat with remaining portions, flouring the surface before rolling out each circle.

11. Place the circles on baking sheets lined with parchment paper.

12. Divide the broccoli mixture into 6 ½-cup portions and place on half of each circle of dough.

13. Dip your finger in water and moisten edges of circles, fold circles in half and crimp the edges to seal.

14. Bake for 15 minutes or until golden brown.

**YIELD: 6 CALZONES**

# Italian-Style Beans and Greens

1 tablespoon extra-virgin olive oil

1/2 cup finely chopped red onion

1 teaspoon sea salt

1 teaspoon red pepper flakes

4 cloves garlic, thinly sliced

2 cups sliced shiitake or button mushrooms

1 1/2 cups (15-ounce can) white cannellini beans, rinsed and drained

1/3 cup dry white wine

8 leaves kale, cleaned, stemmed, and cut into thin ribbons

1. Heat a large skillet over medium heat and add the oil. Add the onion, salt, and red pepper flakes and sauté for 4 minutes, stirring occasionally.

2. Add the garlic, mushrooms, and beans, stir, and sauté for 2 more minutes.

3. Add the wine and stir to mix.

4. Add the kale, stir to coat the leaves, and cover. Reduce heat to medium-low and cook for 5 minutes.

5. Remove the cover and allow the mixture to cook for 2 more minutes so that the extra liquid cooks off.

**YIELD: 4 CUPS**

# Mini Pizzas

*Kids love 'em! Try using an opened and cleaned tuna can to cut rounds. If you don't have a cutter, just cut the crusts off.*

| | |
|---|---|
| 4 | slices whole grain spelt or rice bread |
| 2 | tablespoons extra-virgin olive oil |
| ½ | cup pizza or pasta sauce, homemade or unsweetened store-bought |
| ¼ | cup grated or sliced mozzarella-style soy cheese |
| ½ | cup chopped red or green peppers |
| ½ | cup sliced mushrooms |
| 2 | teaspoons fresh oregano |

1. Preheat the oven or toaster oven to 350°F.

2. Using a round cookie cutter, cut one large circle out of the middle of each slice of bread, saving the crusts for bread crumbs in other recipes. Place the bread circles on a baking sheet so that you don't have to move them after the mini pizzas are assembled.

3. Lightly oil the top of the bread and spread 2 tablespoons of sauce onto each slice.

4. Sprinkle with soy cheese, peppers, mushrooms, and oregano.

5. Bake for 5 minutes or until heated through (soy cheese won't melt as completely as regular cheese).

**YIELD: 4 PIZZAS**

# POPEYE'S SPINACH PIE

|       |                                                    |
|------:|----------------------------------------------------|
| 2     | cups spelt white flour                             |
| 3/4   | teaspoon sea salt, divided                         |
| 1/3   | cup + 1 tablespoon extra-virgin olive oil          |
| 1–2   | tablespoons water                                  |
| 1/2   | cup chopped yellow onion                           |
| 1/2   | cup finely shredded red cabbage                    |
| 1/2   | cup chopped zucchini                               |
| 8     | cups (16 ounces) fresh baby spinach, washed and dried |
| 1     | clove garlic, minced                               |
| 1/2   | teaspoon dried marjoram                            |
| 1/2   | teaspoon dried basil                               |
| 1/2   | teaspoon dried thyme                               |
| 1     | teaspoon dried mustard powder                      |
| 1     | teaspoon paprika                                   |
| 1/4   | teaspoon ground red pepper                         |
| 1     | large tomato, cut into 8 half-moon slices          |

1. Preheat oven to 375°F.

2. To prepare the crust, sift the flour and ¼ teaspoon of the salt into a medium mixing bowl. Slowly pour in ⅓ cup of the oil while stirring to form a dough. Do not overmix or the dough will be too tough. Use up to 2 tablespoons of water to help form the dough.

3. Gather the dough into a ball and lightly roll with a rolling pin until it reaches a 9-inch diameter. Press the rolled dough into a 9-inch pie plate. Poke the bottom of the crust all over with a fork. Set aside while preparing the filling.

4. Heat a medium skillet over medium heat and add the remaining 1 tablespoon of oil and the onion. Sauté for 2 minutes, add the cabbage and zucchini, and sauté an additional 5 minutes. Add the spinach and sauté until wilted.

5. Add the garlic, the remaining ½ teaspoon of salt, marjoram, basil, thyme, mustard, paprika, and pepper. Stir well to combine, and sauté for 1 minute.

6. Pour the mixture into the prepared crust.

7. Bake for 35 minutes.

8. Remove pie from the oven and garnish with a ring of tomato slices.

**YIELD: 1 9″ PIE**

# Sang Choy Bow (Chinese Mushroom Rice "Burritos")

| | |
|---|---|
| 1 | tablespoon toasted sesame oil |
| 2 | cups minced shiitake, enoki, or reishi mushrooms |
| 2 | cloves garlic, minced |
| 2 | tablespoons naturally brewed soy sauce (shoyu or wheat-free tamari) |
| 1 | cup cooked leftover whole grain |
| 1 | medium red bell pepper, seeded and chopped |
| 1/4 | cup chopped celery |
| 1 | piece (1") fresh ginger, peeled and finely chopped |
| 1 | tablespoon rice wine vinegar |
| 1–3 | teaspoons chili paste |
| 1 | cup mung bean sprouts |
| 8 | lettuce leaves, washed and dried |

1. Place a large skillet over medium heat and add the oil.

2. Sauté the mushrooms, garlic, and soy sauce for 2 minutes. Add the grain, bell pepper, celery, and ginger. Stir well to combine and cook for 3 minutes.

3. In a small bowl, combine the vinegar and chili paste. Stir well and pour over the cooking vegetables. Mix well to coat the veggies.

4. Toss the bean sprouts with the cooking vegetables, and remove from heat.

5. Fill each lettuce leaf with about 1/4 cup of the mushroom mixture and serve 2 per person.

**YIELD: 2 1/2 CUPS**

# Savory Stuffed Acorn Squash

| | |
|---|---|
| 1 | acorn squash, about 1½ pounds |
| 2 | tablespoons extra-virgin olive oil, divided |
| 1½ | teaspoons sea salt, divided |
| ¼ | teaspoon ground black pepper |
| ¼ | teaspoon paprika |
| 2 | cups vegetable stock |
| 1 | cup millet, rinsed and drained |
| ¼ | cup minced shallots |
| ¼ | cup thinly sliced shiitake mushrooms |
| ¼ | cup cashews |
| ¼ | cup fresh or thawed frozen cranberries |
| 1 | clove garlic, minced |
| 6 | fresh sage leaves, thinly sliced |

1. Preheat oven to 375°F.

2. Cut the acorn squash in half from stem to pointed tip. Use a spoon to scrape out the seeds and strings. Place both halves cut side up on a baking sheet. Drizzle each squash half with 1½ teaspoons oil, and sprinkle with 1 teaspoon of the salt, the pepper, and the paprika.

3. Bake squash until tender, about 30 to 40 minutes.

4. While the squash cooks, bring the stock to a boil in a medium saucepan and add the millet. Cover, reduce heat to simmer, and cook for 30 minutes.

5. Heat a medium skillet over medium heat and add the remaining 1 tablespoon olive oil. Sauté the shallots, mushrooms, and the remaining ½ teaspoon salt for 5 minutes. Add the cashews, cranberries, garlic, and sage and sauté over low heat for another 10 minutes. Remove from heat while the millet finishes cooking.

6. Add the millet to the skillet and stir well to combine. Place the squash face up on a plate and fill each with the cooked grain mixture. Serve hot.

**YIELD: 2 SQUASH HALVES**

# Thai Protein Noodle Salad

½  package firm tofu, rinsed, drained, and cubed, or 1 cup cooked, cubed protein

1  tablespoon toasted sesame oil or extra-virgin olive oil

1  7-ounce package rice noodles

2  green onions, green and white part chopped

1  cup snow pea shoots, mung bean sprouts, or sunflower sprouts, rinsed and dried

1  red bell pepper, seeded and thinly sliced

1  avocado, peeled, pitted, and cubed

3  tablespoons chopped cashews or peanuts

2  tablespoons naturally brewed soy sauce (shoyu or tamari)

1  teaspoon maple syrup

1  clove garlic, crushed

Juice of 1 lime

1  piece (½") fresh ginger, peeled and minced

1  tablespoon natural, sugar-free, salt-free peanut butter

2  tablespoons fresh cilantro leaves

1. If using tofu as the protein source in this recipe, place a large skillet over medium heat and add the oil. Sauté the tofu until lightly browned on all sides, about 5 minutes. Remove the tofu to a plate lined with paper towels to drain any excess oil and set aside.

2. Cook the rice noodles according to the directions on the package, drain, and rinse under cool water to stop the cooking process.

3. In a large mixing bowl, combine the tofu, green onions, snow pea shoots or sprouts, bell pepper, avocado, and cashews or peanuts. Add the rice noodles and gently stir to combine.

4. In a small mixing bowl, whisk together the soy sauce, maple syrup, garlic, lime juice, ginger, and peanut butter. Pour over the vegetables and mix with a large wooden spoon or rubber spatula.

5. Garnish with fresh cilantro and serve.

**YIELD: 10 CUPS**

# Tofu Vegetable Phyllo Tart

1    package (14 ounces) firm tofu, drained, towel dried, and crumbled with your hands

½    cup olives, pitted

¼    cup finely chopped red onion

¼    cup finely chopped Italian (flat-leaf) parsley

3    tablespoons drained capers

1    clove garlic, chopped

1    tablespoon fresh marjoram leaves

1    teaspoon + ¼ cup extra-virgin olive oil

½    teaspoon naturally brewed soy sauce (shoyu or tamari)

    Freshly ground black pepper to taste

12    sheets thawed phyllo dough

1    orange or red bell pepper, seeded and sliced into long crescents

1    green bell pepper, seeded and sliced into long crescents

6    oil-packed sun-dried tomatoes, drained and cut into halves

1. Preheat oven to 400°F.

2. Combine the tofu, olives, onion, parsley, capers, garlic, marjoram, 1 teaspoon of the oil, the soy sauce, and pepper in a food processor and process until smooth and well combined, scraping down sides once or twice. Set aside.

3. Lightly oil a 9" tart pan with olive oil, using a pastry brush.

4. Layer single pieces of phyllo on the tart pan, allowing the edges to hang over the sides, but lightly pressing the phyllo down to contour with the shape of the pan. Lightly brush the top of each layer with the oil, until you have used all 12 sheets of phyllo.

5. Spoon the tofu filling onto the phyllo tart crust, smoothing it out into an even layer. Fold the edges of the overhanging phyllo up to form a little crust around the edges of the tart. Brush the top of the phyllo crust with the remaining oil.

6. Arrange the bell pepper slices in a circular pattern around the tart, and sprinkle with the tomatoes.

7. Bake, covered with foil, for 30 minutes.

8. Remove the foil and bake for another 10 minutes, or until the top of the crust is lightly browned.

9. Allow to cool about 5 minutes and remove from tart form. Serve warm.

**YIELD: 1 9" PIE, SERVES 4**

# Veggie Burgers

*These tasty burgers freeze well when wrapped individually.*

| | |
|---|---|
| ¼ | cup grated yellow onion |
| ¼ | cup grated red or yellow bell pepper |
| 1½ | cups (15-ounce can) cooked lentils, black beans, or kidney beans, drained |
| ½ | cup coarsely chopped sunflower or pumpkin seeds |
| ½ | cup coarsely chopped walnuts, pecans, or cashews |
| 2 | tablespoons shredded carrot |
| 2 | tablespoons shredded celery |
| 2 | cloves garlic, minced |
| 2 | tablespoons fresh parsley |
| 1 | teaspoon extra-virgin olive oil |
| 1 | teaspoon sea salt |
| 1 | teaspoon naturally brewed soy sauce (shoyu or tamari) |
| 1 | teaspoon dried oregano |
| 1 | teaspoon dried basil |
| ½ | teaspoon chili powder |
| ½ | teaspoon curry powder |
| ½ | teaspoon freshly ground black pepper |
| ¼ | teaspoon ground red pepper |

1. Preheat oven to 350°F.

2. Gently squeeze grated onion and bell pepper in a clean paper towel, to remove excess moisture.

3. Combine the onion, bell pepper, lentils or beans, seeds, nuts, carrot, celery, garlic, parsley, oil, salt, soy sauce, oregano, basil, chili powder, curry powder, black pepper, and ground red pepper in a food processor and pulse until mixture is coarse but blended well. You may need to add a little water so the texture is just moist enough to be able to blend in the food processor. (For best flavor, allow the mixture to set at room temperature, covered, for up to 2 hours.)

4. Place a large piece of waxed paper on a baking sheet or cutting board. Pack a ⅓-cup measuring cup with the mixture and scoop onto the waxed paper for a total of 6 scoops. Shape into patties.

5. Lightly oil a baking sheet. Place the baking sheet on top of the patties, and, holding both together, turn over the cutting board or first baking sheet and lift away. Remove the waxed paper. (This technique allows the burgers to hold their shape well.)

6. Bake for 20 minutes.

7. Serve with whole grain mustard on whole grain buns or bread slices.

**YIELD: 6 PATTIES**

# Veggie Loaf

*This recipe freezes well. Allow the loaf to cool completely, wrap in plastic, and freeze.*

|   |   |
|---|---|
| 1 | cup cooked brown rice or other leftover whole grain |
| 1 | cup cooked lentils, brown or red |
| 1 | cup uncooked instant oats |
| 1 | cup finely chopped mushrooms |
| 1 | medium yellow onion, finely chopped |
| 1 | medium carrot, grated on a cheese grater |
| ½ | red bell pepper, chopped |
| ½ | cup finely chopped walnuts |
| ¼ | cup tomato paste |
| ¼ | cup olives, any variety, pitted and chopped fine |
| 3 | tablespoons finely chopped fresh parsley |
| 2 | tablespoons naturally brewed soy sauce (shoyu or tamari) |
| 2 | tablespoons mustard |
| 1 | teaspoon dried thyme |
| 1 | teaspoon dried marjoram |
| 1 | teaspoon dried sage |

1. Preheat oven to 350°F.
2. In a large mixing bowl, combine the rice or other whole grain, lentils, oats, mushrooms, onion, carrot, pepper, walnuts, tomato paste, olives, parsley, soy sauce, mustard, thyme, marjoram, and sage, and mix well.
3. Lightly oil an 8" × 4" loaf pan with extra-virgin olive oil.
4. Fill the loaf pan with the mixture and pack well to press out any air pockets.
5. Bake for 40 minutes, covered. Uncover and bake for another 20 minutes, until lightly browned. Allow to stand at room temperature for 15 minutes before slicing. Use a serrated knife to carefully slice.

**YIELD: 1 LARGE LOAF, SERVES 8**

# WALNUT BURGER PATTIES

*These keep well when individually wrapped and frozen. They are also great as breakfast patties. Simply add sage and thyme and replace the olives and tomatoes with mushrooms.*

| | |
|---|---|
| 2 | tablespoons extra-virgin olive oil |
| 2 | tablespoons brown rice flour or spelt flour |
| 1 | tablespoon naturally brewed soy sauce (shoyu or wheat-free tamari) |
| 1½ | cups warm vegetable stock or plain soy milk |
| 1 | cup rolled oats |
| ½ | cup chopped yellow onion |
| 1 | cup finely chopped walnuts |
| 1 | cup cooked brown rice or other whole grain |
| ½ | cup pitted and chopped olives |
| ½ | cup chopped sun-dried tomatoes |

1. Place a large skillet over medium-low heat. Add the oil, flour, and soy sauce. Whisk well to combine.

2. Whisk in stock or soy milk and cook until thickened, continuing to whisk, about 2 minutes.

3. Remove from heat and add the oats, onion, walnuts, rice or other whole grain, olives, and tomatoes. Stir well to combine and transfer entire contents to a medium mixing bowl. Allow to set at room temperature for 10 minutes, then refrigerate until cool enough to handle, about 20 minutes.

4. Preheat oven to 350°F.

5. Line a baking sheet with parchment paper.

6. Remove the mixture from refrigerator, and scoop ¼ cup of mixture into a patty. Place on the baking sheet, and continue to scoop mixture into patties until done.

7. Bake for 20 minutes, and serve. If freezing, wrap each patty individually in plastic wrap.

**YIELD: 12 PATTIES**

# Avocado Sesame Pasta

| | |
|---|---|
| 4 | ounces rice or mung bean noodles (gluten, dairy, and wheat free!) |
| 1 | ripe avocado, peeled, pitted, and chopped |
| 4 | cherry tomatoes, quartered (about $1/3$ cup) |
| 2 | tablespoons toasted sesame oil |
| 2 | tablespoons freshly squeezed lime juice |
| 1 | tablespoon hulled sesame seeds |
| 2 | teaspoons naturally brewed soy sauce (shoyu or wheat-free tamari) |
| 2 | cloves garlic, crushed |
| $1/4$ | teaspoon red pepper flakes |
| | Fresh cilantro leaves for garnish (optional) |

1. Cook the pasta according to package directions. Rinse in cold water to stop the cooking and set pasta aside in a serving bowl.

2. In a medium mixing bowl, combine the avocado, tomatoes, sesame oil, lime juice, sesame seeds, soy sauce, garlic, and red pepper flakes.

3. Mix with a spoon and pour over the pasta. Garnish with cilantro, if desired.

**YIELD: 4 CUPS**

# Carrot Muffins

|       |                                   |
|-------|-----------------------------------|
| 2     | cups white spelt flour            |
| 1     | cup whole spelt flour             |
| $1^{1}/_{2}$ | teaspoons baking soda       |
| $1^{1}/_{2}$ | teaspoons baking powder     |
| $^{1}/_{2}$  | teaspoon cardamom powder    |
| $^{1}/_{2}$  | teaspoon cinnamon           |
| $^{1}/_{4}$  | teaspoon freshly ground nutmeg |
| $^{1}/_{2}$  | cup unsweetened applesauce  |
| 1     | cup water                         |
| $^{1}/_{3}$  | cup olive or unrefined coconut oil |
| 1     | tablespoon vanilla extract        |
| 2     | tablespoons apple cider vinegar   |
| $^{1}/_{4}$  | teaspoon sea salt           |
|       | Zest of 1 orange                  |
| $1^{1}/_{2}$ | cups grated carrot          |
| $^{1}/_{2}$  | cup unsweetened shredded coconut |
| 1     | cup maple syrup                   |
| 1     | cup raisins                       |

1. Preheat oven to 325°F.

2. In a large mixing bowl, sift together the white spelt flour, whole spelt flour, baking soda, baking powder, cardamom, cinnamon, and nutmeg. Stir to combine and set aside.

3. In a blender, combine the applesauce, water, oil, vanilla, vinegar, salt, orange zest, carrot, coconut, and maple syrup. Blend until well combined.

4. Fold the wet ingredients into the dry, add the raisins, and stir until just mixed.

5. Pour ¼-cup scoops of batter into oiled muffin pans and bake for 20 minutes.

**YIELD: 24 3" MUFFINS**

# Coconut Curry Rice

 2 cups brown rice, rinsed and drained

 1 can (14 ounces) unsweetened coconut milk

 2 cups filtered water

 1 tablespoon curry powder

 1 teaspoon sea salt

 1/2 teaspoon ground red pepper

 1/2 cup raisins

1. Combine the rice, coconut milk, water, curry powder, salt, and pepper in a 4 quart pot and stir well.

2. Place over medium-high heat, cover, and bring to a boil.

3. When rice begins to boil, turn the heat down to low and allow to simmer for 45 to 50 minutes.

4. When the rice is cooked through, add the raisins and stir to incorporate, then cover and allow to sit for 10 minutes.

5. Serve hot or cold.

**YIELD: 7 CUPS**

# Corny Corn Bread

*Cooking in cast-iron skillets has been known to add vital iron to meals, which is good for women and those with anemia.*

| | |
|---|---|
| 1 | cup stone-ground cornmeal |
| 1/2 | teaspoon sea salt |
| 1/2 | teaspoon baking soda |
| 1 | cup plain soy milk, almond milk, or water |
| 1 | tablespoon fresh lemon juice |
| 1 | heaping tablespoon soy flour mixed with 2 tablespoons water, or 1 serving egg substitute |
| 1 | cup fresh or frozen and thawed corn kernels |
| 1 | tablespoon extra-virgin olive oil |

1. Heat oven to 450°F.
2. Heat a 12-inch cast-iron skillet over low heat while you mix the batter.
3. In a medium mixing bowl, combine the cornmeal, salt, and baking soda. Stir well to blend.
4. In a small mixing bowl, combine the milk or water, lemon juice, and soy flour mixture or egg substitute. Stir in the corn kernels.
5. Pour the milk mixture into the cornmeal and stir until just combined.
6. Add the olive oil to the skillet and tilt all around to coat the bottom well.
7. Pour the bread mixture into the skillet and place on the middle rack in the oven.
8. Bake for 15 minutes, or until a knife poked into the center of the bread comes out clean.

**YIELD: 1 12" ROUND**

# CREAMY TOMATO MILLET WITH FRESH HERBS

| | |
|---|---|
| 2½ | cups filtered water |
| 1 | cup millet, rinsed and drained |
| 2 | teaspoons sea salt, divided |
| ¼ | cup extra-virgin olive oil |
| ½ | vegetable bouillon cube |
| 2 | pounds ripe plum tomatoes (about 14), chopped and seeded |
| ¼ | teaspoon freshly ground black pepper |
| ½ | cup plain soy milk or fresh nut milk |
| 2 | teaspoons fresh basil, finely sliced |
| 1 | teaspoon fresh rosemary, minced |
| 1 | teaspoon fresh sage, minced |
| 1 | teaspoon fresh Italian (flat-leaf) parsley |

1. Bring the water to a boil in a 4 quart pot and add the millet and 1 teaspoon of the salt. Cover, lower heat to a simmer, and cook for 30 minutes, until the water is completely absorbed. Fluff with a fork and set aside.

2. Place a large skillet over medium heat and add the oil. Add the bouillon cube and stir with a wooden spoon until the cube has completely dissolved, about 1 minute.

3. Add the tomatoes, and season with the remaining 1 teaspoon of salt and the pepper. Cook, stirring often, for 5 minutes.

4. Pour in the milk and cook, stirring frequently, until the liquid has reduced by half, about 15 minutes. Remove the skillet from the heat and set aside.

5. Toss the millet with the sauce and the basil, rosemary, sage, and parsley. Serve hot.

**YIELD: 5 CUPS**

# Mushroom Barley Pilaf

| | |
|---|---|
| 3 | cups unsalted vegetable stock |
| 1 | cup raw pearled barley, rinsed and drained |
| 3/4 | teaspoon sea salt |
| 2 | tablespoons extra-virgin olive oil |
| 1 | cup chopped yellow onion |
| 1 | celery stalk, thinly sliced |
| 2 | cloves garlic, minced |
| 1 | teaspoon dry oregano |
| 1/2 | teaspoon freshly ground black pepper |
| 2 | cups shiitake mushrooms, chopped |
| 2 | tablespoons chopped fresh parsley |
| 2 | tablespoons naturally brewed soy sauce (shoyu or tamari) |

1. In a 4 quart pot, bring the vegetable stock to a boil, add the barley and ¼ teaspoon of the salt, cover, reduce heat to a simmer, and cook for about 50 minutes, or until the liquid is gone.

2. Place a large skillet over medium heat and add the oil. Add the onion, celery, and the remaining ½ teaspoon of salt and sauté for 5 minutes, or until the onion becomes translucent. Add the garlic, oregano, pepper, and mushrooms. Sauté for another 8 minutes.

3. Add the cooked barley and stir well to combine. Stir in the parsley and soy sauce. Serve hot.

**YIELD: 6 CUPS**

# Parsley, Sage, Rosemary, and Thyme Rice

2½ cups filtered water or unsalted vegetable stock

1 cup brown rice, rinsed and drained

1 teaspoon sea salt

½ cup chopped onion

1 teaspoon fresh parsley

1 teaspoon fresh sage

1 teaspoon fresh rosemary

1 teaspoon fresh thyme

1. In a 4 quart pot, bring the water or stock to a boil. Add the rice, salt, and onion. Stir to dissolve any clumps and cover.

2. Cook for 45 to 60 minutes, or until the rice is cooked and all the liquid has evaporated.

3. Stir in the parsley, sage, rosemary, and thyme and allow to sit for a few minutes so that the aromas of the herbs begin to appear. Serve hot.

**YIELD: 4 CUPS**


# Polenta

2 cups water

1 teaspoon sea salt

1 cup cornmeal

¼ cup chopped yellow or white onion

1. Bring the water to a boil in a small saucepan.

2. Add the sea salt and slowly pour the cornmeal into the water while whisking continuously to avoid lumps.

3. Add the onion, stir to combine, and cover. Turn heat to lowest setting and cook for 15 minutes.

4. Serve with chili or pasta sauce.

**YIELD: 2½ CUPS**

# Quinoa Pilaf

| | |
|---|---|
| 2 | tablespoons extra-virgin olive oil |
| ½ | cup chopped red onion |
| 1 | cup shredded carrot |
| 1 | cup quinoa |
| 2 | cloves garlic, minced |
| 2 | cups filtered water |
| 2 | teaspoons naturally brewed soy sauce (shoyu or tamari) |
| ½ | cup fresh or thawed frozen peas |

1. Heat a 4 quart pot over medium heat.

2. Add the oil and sauté the onion, carrot, and quinoa until the quinoa begins to turn light brown and lets off a nutty smell.

3. Add the garlic, water, and soy sauce.

4. Stir well and cover. Bring to a boil and reduce heat to a simmer. Cook until all the water is absorbed and the quinoa is light and fluffy, about 20 minutes.

5. Add the peas and stir to combine. Cover, remove from heat, and allow to sit for 5 minutes before serving.

**YIELD: 4½ CUPS**

# SPICY RED BEANS AND SAVORY RICE

1⅓ cups cooked or 1 15-ounce can red kidney
beans, drained, sorted, and rinsed

6 cups filtered water, divided

1 piece (2") kombu

4 tablespoons extra-virgin olive oil, divided

2 cups chopped red onion, divided

3 cloves garlic, minced

2 bay leaves

1 tablespoon maple syrup

1 vegetable bouillon cube

1 teaspoon dried oregano

1 teaspoon crushed red pepper flakes

1½ teaspoons sea salt, divided

1 cup brown rice

1 cup chopped carrot (about 2 medium carrots)

1 cup chopped celery (about 2 medium stalks)

1 cup seeded and chopped red bell pepper

½ cup fresh corn kernels or thawed frozen kernels

2 tablespoons chopped fresh parsley

1. Place the beans, 2 cups of the water, and the kombu in a medium saucepan over high heat. Cover and bring to a boil. Lower the temperature to a simmer and cook for 20 minutes. Remove the kombu and discard it. Remove the saucepan from the heat and set aside.

2. Lightly coat a large Dutch oven with 1 tablespoon of the oil and place over medium heat until hot. Add 1 cup of the onion and the garlic and sauté until tender, about 3 minutes.

3. Drain and add the beans, 2 cups of the water, the bay leaves, maple syrup, bouillon cube, oregano, red pepper flakes, and ½ teaspoon of the salt. Cover, bring to a boil, and reduce heat to a simmer. Cook for 30 minutes or until beans are tender.

4. While the beans are cooking, prepare the rice. Pour the remaining 2 cups water in a 4 quart pot, cover, and place over high heat. When boiling, add the rice and ½ teaspoon of the salt. Cover, reduce heat to a simmer, and cook for 45 to 55 minutes.

5. Place a large skillet over medium heat and add the remaining 3 tablespoons of oil. Add the remaining 1 cup of onion, the carrot, celery, bell pepper, corn, and the remaining ½ teaspoon salt. Sauté for 10 minutes, stirring often, and set aside.

6. Toss the vegetables with the rice. Add the parsley. Serve the kidney beans over the rice.

**YIELD: 7½ CUPS**

# Riso di Basilico

*A healthy take on a traditional Italian pasta dish.*

| | |
|---|---|
| 2 | cups (2 ounces) loosely packed fresh basil leaves, carefully washed and dried |
| 2 | tablespoons pine nuts |
| 2 | cloves garlic, minced |
| 2 | tablespoons white or yellow miso paste |
| ½ | cup extra-virgin olive oil |
| 6 | cups cooked brown rice or other whole grain |

1. Put the basil, pine nuts, garlic, and miso paste into a food processor and begin processing. Slowly add the oil in a fine stream until smooth and creamy. You may need to scrape the sides of the processor down to make sure the mixture is completely blended.

2. Transfer the mixture to a large bowl and stir in the rice or other whole grain.

3. Serve cold as a salad or hot as a side dish.

**YIELD: 7 CUPS**

# CITRUS AVOCADO PESTO

*Works as a wonderful vegetable dip for chips, crackers, bread, or crudité.*

| | |
|---|---|
| 3 | medium, very ripe avocados, peeled, pitted, and chopped |
| 2 | tablespoons fresh lemon juice |
| 1 | tablespoon fresh orange juice |
| 1 | tablespoon fresh lime juice |
| 3 | cloves garlic, minced |
| 1 | cup packed fresh cilantro leaves |
| 1 | teaspoon sea salt |

1. Combine the avocados, lemon juice, orange juice, lime juice, garlic, cilantro, and salt in a blender and blend until smooth.

2. Store in a glass container with plastic wrap pressed closely to the top of the pesto to prevent browning.

**YIELD: 2 CUPS**

# CRANBERRY RELISH

*An "old family recipe" updated for healthier holidays.*

| | |
|---|---|
| 2 | cups pure maple syrup |
| 1 | package frozen or fresh cranberries |
| 1½ | cups golden seedless raisins |
| ½ | cup apple cider vinegar |
| 1 | large orange (juice, pulp, and grated zest) |
| 1 | teaspoon cinnamon |
| 1 | teaspoon ground cloves |
| 1 | teaspoon ground ginger |

1. Combine the maple syrup, cranberries, raisins, vinegar, orange, cinnamon, cloves, and ginger in a large saucepan, cover, bring to a slow boil, and cook for 10 to 15 minutes. You will hear the cranberries popping. Once the popping stops, lift the cover and stir once or twice.

2. Serve chilled or hot. Store in the refrigerator in an airtight container for 2 to 3 weeks.

**YIELD: 4 CUPS**

# CURRY DRESSING

*Use over salads, vegetables, beans, grains, or protein dishes.*

| | |
|---|---|
| 1 | cup coconut oil or extra-virgin olive oil |
| 3 | tablespoons apple cider vinegar |
| 1 | tablespoon + 1 teaspoon curry powder |
| ½ | teaspoon freshly ground pepper |

1. Whisk the oil, vinegar, curry powder, and pepper together in a small bowl until well combined. Keeps refrigerated in an airtight glass container for 1 month.

**YIELD: 1¼ CUPS**

# Dill Tofu Dip

*Great with raw carrot sticks!*

| | |
|---|---|
| 1 | 14-ounce block soft tofu, drained and patted dry |
| ¼ | cup fresh lemon juice |
| 3 | tablespoons finely minced yellow onion |
| 2 | cloves garlic, minced |
| 2 | tablespoons chopped fresh dill |
| 2 | tablespoons chickpea miso |
| 2 | tablespoons water |
| 1 | tablespoon balsamic vinegar |
| ½ | teaspoon sea salt |
| | Freshly ground black pepper to taste |

1. Put the tofu, lemon juice, onion, garlic, dill, miso, water, vinegar, salt, and pepper into a blender and blend well. Add more water, if necessary, to reach desired consistency. Allow the flavors to marry in the refrigerator for at least 2 hours before serving.

**YIELD: 2 CUPS**

# Easy, Best Salad Dressing

| 8 | tablespoons extra-virgin olive oil or flaxseed oil |
|---|---|
| 4 | tablespoons fresh lemon juice |
| 4 | teaspoons Dijon mustard |
| 2 | teaspoons sea salt |
| 1 | teaspoon maple syrup |
| 1/2 | teaspoon freshly ground black pepper |
| | Fresh herbs, minced garlic, or chopped capers (optional) |

1. Combine the oil, lemon juice, mustard, salt, maple syrup, and pepper in a bowl and whisk together. For an extra kick, whisk in fresh herbs, garlic, or capers. Serve over salads or steamed veggies.

2. Store in an airtight glass container in the refrigerator. Remove from refrigerator and allow to sit at room temperature for 30 minutes before shaking and serving.

**YIELD: 2/3 CUP**

# Easy Chutney

*Use this rich mixture to spice up bean and rice dishes, or spread it on a protein dish for a quick variation.*

| 2 | tablespoons extra-virgin olive oil |
|---|---|
| 1 | cup chopped red onion |
| 1 | cup raisins, pulse until fine in a food processor or chop coarsely |
| 1/2 | teaspoon sea salt |
| 1/4 | teaspoon cinnamon |
| 1/4 | teaspoon red pepper flakes |
| | Dash of freshly ground black pepper |

1. Heat a medium skillet over medium heat and add the oil. Sauté the onions until they just begin to brown.

2. Add the raisins, salt, cinnamon, red pepper flakes, and black pepper. Continue to sauté for 5 more minutes, stirring often.

3. Serve hot or cold. Keep refrigerated in an airtight glass container for up to 2 weeks.

**YIELD: 1³/₄ CUPS**

## GOMASIO

*This traditional Japanese flavoring is a great replacement for regular table salt.*

- 1 cup sesame seeds
- 1 tablespoon sea salt
- 2 tablespoons crushed nori (optional)

1. Place a medium skillet over medium heat and dry-toast the sesame seeds until they begin to let off a nutty aroma, or begin to turn golden brown. Do not allow the seeds to burn.

2. Pour the seeds, salt, and nori (if using) into a mortar and pestle or blender and grind the seeds using gentle pressure until the seeds become half-crushed.

3. Store in an airtight glass jar in the refrigerator.

**YIELD: 1 CUP**

# Guacamole

4   medium, very ripe Haas avocados, peeled, pitted, and finely chopped

½   cup quartered cherry tomatoes (about 6 tomatoes)

¼   small red onion, chopped

¼   cup chopped fresh cilantro

1   tablespoon fresh lime juice

1   clove garlic, minced

1   teaspoon sea salt

1. In a large bowl, mash the avocados, tomatoes, onion, cilantro, lime juice, garlic, and salt with a potato masher until well combined.

**YIELD: 3½ CUPS**

# Homemade Miso Tofu Cheese Spread

1   block firm tofu

1   cup miso paste, any flavor

1. Line a sieve with paper towels and place the tofu inside. Pull up the paper towels to cover the tofu, and weight with a can laid on its side or two or three stacked bowls. Allow the tofu to drain for 15 minutes, or until about ⅓ cup of the liquid has drained out.

2. Place 2 tablespoons of the miso on a small plate and smooth it out to roughly the size of the largest side of the tofu. Place the drained tofu on the miso and spread the remaining miso paste on all surfaces of the tofu to completely cover.

3. Lightly wrap the tofu with plastic wrap and refrigerate for 24 hours.

4. Unwrap the tofu and gently scrape off the miso paste. The tofu will have taken on the color and flavor of the miso, and it can now be used as a delicious spread for vegetables or crackers or as a substitute for the ricotta cheese in lasagna.

**YIELD: 3 CUPS**

# HOMEMADE NUT BUTTER

*Raw or roasted nuts can be used for this recipe. Free of hydrogenated fat and added sugar, this recipe is easy and delicious! Roasted nuts really enhance the flavor and aroma of the butter.*

- **4**   **cups raw or roasted\* nuts (almonds, peanuts, Brazil nuts, cashews, hazelnuts, macadamia nuts, or pecans)**
- **1**   **teaspoon sea salt**
- **2**   **tablespoons extra-virgin olive oil or unrefined nontoasted sesame oil**
- **2**   **tablespoons finely chopped nuts (optional)**

1. Combine the nuts and salt in a blender or food processor fit with a blade and pulse until the nuts are finely ground.

2. Add the oil and continue to pulse until the butter is creamy. You may need to scrape down the sides of the blender or processor with a rubber spatula. Add more oil as necessary.

3. For a chunkier version, stir in 2 tablespoons finely chopped nuts.

4. Store, tightly covered in a glass container, in the refrigerator.

**YIELD: 2 CUPS**

**\*Note:** *To roast nuts, spread them in a thin layer, not crowding each other, on an unoiled baking sheet for 15 minutes at 325°F. Check on the nuts and stir them after approximately 8 minutes for evenly roasted nuts.*

# KETCHUP

*Preservative- and corn syrup–free!*

| | |
|---|---|
| 1 | 6-ounce can tomato paste |
| 1/4 | cup filtered water |
| 1/4 | cup maple or brown rice syrup |
| 2 | tablespoons cider vinegar |
| 1/2 | teaspoon salt |
| 1/2 | teaspoon ground cumin |
| 1/4 | teaspoon dry mustard |
| 1/4 | teaspoon ground cinnamon |
| 1/8 | teaspoon ground cloves |

1. Blend the tomato paste, water, syrup, vinegar, salt, cumin, mustard, cinnamon, and cloves together in a blender until very smooth.

2. Refrigerate in a tightly sealed container. Will keep for 1 month.

**YIELD: 1 CUP**

# LEMONY GARLIC MUSTARD SALAD DRESSING

| | |
|---|---|
| 1/2 | cup extra-virgin olive oil or flaxseed oil |
| 5 | tablespoons freshly squeezed lemon juice (about 3 lemons) |
| 2 | cloves garlic, minced |
| 1/4 | teaspoon sea salt |
| 2 | teaspoons stone-ground mustard |

1. Combine the oil, lemon juice, garlic, salt, and mustard in a bowl and whisk together for 1 minute.

2. Use on salad or vegetables right away, or refrigerate in an airtight glass jar for up to 2 weeks.

**YIELD: 1 CUP**

# Red Raspberry Jam

4   cups red raspberries, fresh or unsweetened
    thawed frozen berries (juice reserved)

1   cup brown rice syrup or maple syrup

¼   cup strained fresh lemon juice

1. Sort through raspberries and remove any that are moldy. Rinse
   and drain well.

2. Combine the berries, syrup, and lemon juice in a medium stainless steel pot and place over medium heat. Stir well and bring the
   mixture to a low boil. Remove from heat.

3. Allow the mixture to cool for 5 minutes. Pour into a blender.
   Blend well and store in airtight glass containers. Will keep for up
   to 2 weeks without canning.

**YIELD: 3½ CUPS**

# Sassy Homemade Applesauce

| | |
|---|---|
| 2 | pounds apples |
| 1 | tablespoon fresh lemon juice |
| 1 | cup orange juice |
| ¼–½ | cup maple or brown rice syrup, depending on sweetness of apples |
| 1 | teaspoon ginger juice* |
| 1 | cinnamon stick |
| 2 | fresh cloves |

1. Peel, core, and chop the apples into ½" slices, tossing them with the lemon juice to prevent discoloration.

2. Place the apples and the orange juice, syrup, ginger juice, cinnamon stick, and cloves in a large, heavy pot. Cover and bring to a low boil. Reduce heat to a simmer, and cook until apples are tender, about 10 to 15 minutes. Uncover the pot and cook 5 minutes more.

3. Remove the pot from the heat and discard the cinnamon stick and cloves. Using a potato masher, mash the apples with the cooking juices. Cool to room temperature, place in an airtight container, and refrigerate.

**YIELD: 4 CUPS**

*Note:* To make ginger juice, shred a 2-inch piece of fresh ginger on the smallest holes of a cheese grater. Gather all of the pulp and squeeze out the juice into a small cup or bowl.

# Savory Seeds

| | |
|---|---|
| 2 | cups raw pumpkin seeds |
| 2 | tablespoons naturally brewed soy sauce (shoyu or tamari) |
| ½ | teaspoon ground red pepper |

1. Preheat oven to 325°F.

2. In a medium mixing bowl, combine the seeds, soy sauce, and pepper. Allow to sit for 20 minutes at room temperature.

3. Pour the soaked seeds onto a large baking sheet lined with foil.

4. Bake the seeds for 8 to 10 minutes, or until they start to become fragrant, stirring occasionally.

5. Allow to cool and serve.

**YIELD: 2 CUPS**

# SUN-DRIED TOMATO SPREAD (TAPENADE)

*A wonderful way to spice up steamed vegetables or grain and bean dishes.*

| | |
|---|---|
| 1 | cup oil-packed sun-dried tomatoes, drained, or 1 cup dried, reconstituted in hot water for 15 minutes, drained |
| 6 | tablespoons extra-virgin olive oil + additional for storing |
| 2 | cloves garlic, minced |
| 1 | tablespoon fresh basil |
| 1 | teaspoon fresh oregano |
| 1 | teaspoon chopped fresh rosemary |
| 1 | teaspoon fresh lemon juice |
| ½ | teaspoon sea salt |

1. Combine the tomatoes, oil, garlic, basil, oregano, rosemary, lemon juice, and salt in a food processor fitted with a blade. Process until pureed and well incorporated. You may need to scrape the sides down a couple of times.

2. Store in a clean glass airtight container and top with a little more olive oil. Will keep refrigerated for up to 1 month.

**YIELD: 1 CUP**

# Sweet and Sour Sauce

*A tasty sauce for protein dishes and a great replacement for those sugary, store-bought varieties.*

- 1 cup unsalted vegetable stock
- ¼ cup maple syrup or brown rice syrup
- ¼ cup apple cider vinegar
- 1 tablespoon kudzu dissolved in ¼ cup filtered water
- 1 tablespoon naturally brewed soy sauce (shoyu or tamari)

1. Combine the stock, syrup, and vinegar in a 4 quart pot over medium heat.

2. Bring to a boil and stir in the kudzu and soy sauce.

3. Lower heat to a simmer and cook for 5 minutes.

4. Use over protein, grains, beans, and vegetable dishes.

**YIELD: 1½ CUPS**

# Tofu "Ricotta"

| | |
|---|---|
| 1 | package (16 ounces) firm tofu, rinsed and drained |
| 1/4 | cup packed, shredded fresh basil |
| 1/4 | cup chopped fresh Italian (flat-leaf) parsley |
| 2 | tablespoons finely chopped red onion |
| 2 | tablespoons fresh thyme leaves |
| 2 | cloves garlic, minced |
| 1 | tablespoon extra-virgin olive oil |
| 1 | teaspoon fresh lemon juice |
| 1/2 | teaspoon sea salt |
| 1 | teaspoon freshly ground black pepper |

1. Combine the tofu, basil, parsley, onion, thyme, garlic, oil, lemon juice, salt, and pepper in the bowl of a food processor, and pulse several times until well blended. The mixture should be crumbly.

2. Use as a sandwich spread, vegetable dip, or lasagna filling.

**YIELD: 2 CUPS**

# Easy Bein' Green Sauté

*Serve with beans and grains for a wonderful, complete meal.*

| | |
|---|---|
| 2 | tablespoon extra-virgin olive oil |
| ½ | cup chopped red onion |
| 2 | cloves garlic, sliced |
| 1 | teaspoon sea salt |
| 1 | head greens, washed and lightly shaken and chopped (kale, collard greens, chard, or bok choy) |
| 1-2 | tablespoons sliced olives, sliced reconstituted sun-dried tomatoes, or capers (optional) |

1. Heat a large skillet over medium heat and add the oil. Sauté the onion, garlic, and salt for 1 minute, stirring often.

2. Add the greens and stir well to coat the leaves with oil.

3. Cover with the lid, reduce heat to low, and allow greens to steam for 3 minutes.

4. After 3 minutes, the greens should begin to turn bright green. Stop cooking now or, for more tender leaves, continue to cook for a few more minutes.

5. Add olives, tomatoes, or capers for extra kick!

**YIELD: 4 CUPS**

# Falafel Chickpea Patties

*Great as sandwiches or served with hummus and olives.*

| | |
|---|---|
| 3 | cups cooked, dried chickpeas, or 2 16-ounce cans, drained and lightly rinsed |
| 3 | tablespoons fresh lemon juice |
| 2 | cloves garlic, minced |
| ½ | cup tahini (sesame seed butter) |
| ½ | cup whole spelt flour |
| ⅓ | cup extra-virgin olive oil |
| 2 | tablespoons filtered water |
| 2 | teaspoons sea salt |
| 2 | teaspoons Tabasco sauce |
| 1 | teaspoon ground cumin |
| ⅛ | teaspoon ground red pepper |

1. Preheat oven to 350°F.

2. Place the chickpeas, lemon juice, and garlic in a food processor. Process until the beans are smooth. You may need to stop, scrape down the sides with a spatula, and process again.

3. Add the tahini, flour, oil, water, salt, Tabasco sauce, cumin, and pepper, and process until well combined. (Add more flour if the mixture is too loose.)

4. Scoop the falafel mixture in ¼-cup scoops and place on a baking sheet lined with parchment paper.

5. Bake for 20 to 25 minutes, until baked through. Serve warm or cold.

**YIELD: 14 PATTIES**

# Italian-Style Crispy Cauliflower

    1/4   cup finely chopped pitted olives, such as
          kalamata or Greek

     2    tablespoons capers, rinsed and drained

     3    tablespoons extra-virgin olive oil, divided

     1    tablespoon red wine vinegar

    1/4   cup finely chopped red onion

     1    clove garlic, minced

     4    cups cauliflower florets (about 1 small head
          or half of a large head)

    1/4   cup filtered water

    1/4   cup chopped fresh Italian (flat-leaf) parsley

          Salt and pepper, to taste

1. In a small bowl, stir together the olives, capers, 2 tablespoons of
   the oil, and the vinegar. Set aside.

2. Heat a large skillet over medium-high heat and add the remaining
   1 tablespoon of oil. Add the onion and sauté for 3 minutes. Add
   the garlic and stir to combine.

3. Add the cauliflower and water to the skillet, stir, and cover. Cook
   for 10 minutes, stirring occasionally.

4. Uncover and sauté cauliflower until tender and browned, but not
   too soft, about 5 minutes. Transfer cauliflower to a large bowl
   and toss with the olive mixture and parsley until well coated.
   Season with salt and pepper to taste.

5. Serve hot.

**YIELD: 4 CUPS**

# Mashed Sweet Potatoes

    1 1/2  pounds sweet potatoes, peeled and cut into
           2" chunks

     1     tablespoon flaxseed oil

     1     tablespoon maple syrup

    1/4    teaspoon chili powder

¼ teaspoon sea salt

2 tablespoons slivered almonds, toasted (optional)

1. Bring a 6 to 8 quart pot of water to a boil and cook the sweet potatoes for about 12 minutes, or until soft.

2. Drain and transfer the sweet potatoes to a large mixing bowl. Add the oil, maple syrup, chili powder, and salt and mash well with a potato masher.

3. Top with toasted almonds, if desired, and serve hot.

**YIELD: 5 CUPS**

## Nori or Lettuce Leaf Wrap-Ups

*Nori, or sushi paper, can be found in Asian markets and health food stores.*

8 whole nori sheets or large lettuce leaves

1 cup guacamole

1 cup grated carrot

½ cucumber, cut in half horizontally, seeded, and sliced into ¼" slices

1 cup sprouts (alfalfa, broccoli, or mung bean)

1 cooked chicken breast, cooled and shredded, or 1 cooked salmon fillet, cooled and flaked, or 1 package (14 ounces) firm tofu, cut in 1" strips, sautéed, and cooled (optional)

1. Place one nori sheet, shiny side down, on a clean, dry surface. If using lettuce leaves instead, wash and dry whole leaves and cut off the bottom 1-inch of stem.

2. Drop 2 tablespoons of guacamole onto the nori sheet or lettuce leaf. Spread the guacamole across the sheet using the back of a spoon, being careful not to tear the sheet or leaf.

3. Spread 2 tablespoons each of the carrot, cucumber, and sprouts across the guacamole.

4. Lay 2 tablespoons of the chicken, salmon, or tofu (if using) across the vegetables and roll up the nori or lettuce leaf like a burrito, gently rolling one side over until the wrap is complete.

**YIELD: 8 ROLLS**

# Overnight Slaw

*A simple pickle recipe for vegetables to help aid digestion.*

| | |
|---|---|
| 4 | cups shredded red or green cabbage |
| 1/2 | cup chopped yellow or white onion |
| 1/2 | cup shredded carrot |
| 1/4 | cup chopped red pepper |
| 2/3 | cup apple cider vinegar |
| 1/2 | cup extra-virgin olive oil |
| 1 | tablespoon maple or brown rice syrup |
| 1/2 | teaspoon sea salt |
| 1/4 | teaspoon dried basil |
| 1/4 | teaspoon dried dill |
| 1/4 | teaspoon dried thyme |

1. Combine the cabbage, onion, carrot, and pepper in a large mixing bowl.

2. Whisk the vinegar, oil, syrup, salt, basil, dill, and thyme together in a medium mixing bowl. Pour over the vegetables and mix well with a large spoon.

3. Cover the vegetable bowl with plastic wrap and refrigerate for at least 8 hours or up to 2 days.

4. Remove the vegetables from the refrigerator, stir, drain the excess liquid, and serve.

**YIELD: 5 CUPS**

# Roasted Winter Squash Smiles

| | |
|---|---|
| 1 | kabocha or other hearty winter squash |
| 1–2 | tablespoons extra-virgin olive oil |
| 1/2 | teaspoon sea salt |
| 1 | tablespoon fresh sage |

1. Preheat oven to 400°F.
2. Rinse off the squash and pat dry.
3. Cut the squash in half and scoop out the seeds (save the seeds for roasting later or planting for your own squash sprouts!).
4. Cut the squash halves into 10 equal slices, each about 1 inch thick.
5. Place the slices on a baking sheet and drizzle the oil and sprinkle the salt over the slices. Make sure the slices are not overlapping, but equally spread out over the baking sheet.
6. Bake for 30 minutes, turning the slices once. In the last 5 minutes, sprinkle the squash smiles with the sage.

**YIELD: 10 SLICES**

## Spicy Sweet Potato Fries

| | |
|---|---|
| 2 | large potatoes, washed, scrubbed, dried, and cut into 1/2" "fries" |
| 1 | medium sweet potato, washed, scrubbed, dried, and cut into 1/2" "fries" |
| 2 | tablespoons extra-virgin olive oil |
| 2 | teaspoons chili powder |
| 2 | teaspoons salt |
| 2 | teaspoons pepper |
| 1 | teaspoon dry oregano |
| 1 | teaspoon dry mustard |
| 1 | teaspoon paprika |

1. Preheat the oven to 425°F.
2. Combine the potatoes, sweet potato, oil, chili powder, salt, pepper, oregano, mustard, and paprika on a large baking sheet, and toss well to coat all fries evenly.
3. Bake for 25 to 30 minutes, until fries are tender, tossing after about 15 minutes.

**YIELD: 5 CUPS**

# Veggie Pâté

*An excellent spread for sandwiches and crackers, or dip for raw veggie sticks!*

| | |
|---|---|
| 1 | cup raw sunflower seeds |
| 1 | cup freshly cooked lentils or 1 cup canned lentils, drained |
| 1/2 | cup grated zucchini |
| 1/2 | cup grated carrot |
| 1/2 | cup grated red onion |
| 1/3 | cup hulled sesame seeds |
| 1/3 | cup extra-virgin olive oil |
| 2 | cloves garlic, minced |
| 2 | tablespoons naturally brewed soy sauce (shoyu or wheat-free tamari) |
| 1 | tablespoon filtered water |
| 1/2 | teaspoon dried basil |
| 1/2 | teaspoon dried thyme |
| 1/2 | teaspoon dried sage |
| 1/8 | teaspoon freshly ground nutmeg |

1. Pulse the sunflower seeds in a food processor until well ground.

2. Add the lentils, zucchini, carrot, onion, sesame seeds, oil, garlic, soy sauce, water, basil, thyme, sage, and nutmeg. Process until well combined.

3. Using a rubber spatula, scrape the pâté into a medium mixing bowl.

4. Cover with plastic wrap and place in the refrigerator. Allow the flavors to marry for at least 1 hour, stir, and serve.

**YIELD: 4 1/4 CUPS**

# Baked Apples

*A nice, easy substitute for apple pie!*

| | |
|---|---|
| 2 | apples, washed, dried, and cored |
| 1/2 | teaspoon cinnamon |
| 1/4 | teaspoon fresh nutmeg |
| 1 | tablespoon maple syrup or honey |
| 1/4 | cup chopped pecans, walnuts, or other nuts (optional) |

1. Preheat oven to 350°F.

2. Cut the apples in half and place in an oven-proof casserole dish.

3. Whisk the cinnamon, nutmeg, and maple syrup or honey together and pour over the apples. Sprinkle the apples with nuts, if using.

4. Bake, covered with aluminum foil, for 20 minutes.

5. Remove the foil, and bake uncovered for another 5 to 10 minutes. Serve hot.

**YIELD: 2 SERVINGS**

# BERRY FUDGY-CICLES

12   ounces silken tofu, rinsed and patted dry

½   cup maple or brown rice syrup

¼   cup cocoa powder

1   tablespoon extra-virgin olive oil

1   teaspoon vanilla extract

    Pinch sea salt

4   strawberries, washed, stemmed, dried, and sliced into quarters

1. Add the tofu, syrup, cocoa, oil, vanilla, and salt to a blender and blend well until smooth and creamy.

2. Pour mixture into popsicle molds or ice cube trays.

3. Drop the strawberry slices into each mold. Insert clean popsicle sticks or toothpicks for handles.

4. Freeze for at least 3 hours to ensure the popsicles are completely frozen.

*Optional method:*

1. Complete step 1.

2. Pour mixture into 8, 2-ounce Dixie cups.

3. Place cups in freezer and insert popsicle sticks into mixture after 20 minutes so that the sticks stand up on their own. Freeze for at least 3 hours.

**YIELD: 8 2-OUNCE POPSICLES**

# Chocolate Anthills

| | |
|---|---|
| 1 | cup grain-sweetened chocolate chips (Sunspire makes a great version.) |
| 1/2 | cup unsweetened, natural nut butter (almond and peanut are great) |
| 2 | cups cooked, cooled brown rice |
| 1/2 | cup chopped nuts |

1. In a medium saucepan, slowly melt and mix the chocolate chips and nut butter together over low heat until well combined. Remove from heat.

2. Add the rice and nuts.

3. Stir together until completely mixed.

4. Line a baking sheet with waxed paper. Drop heaping tablespoons of the mixture onto the baking sheet, and place in the refrigerator to set for 30 minutes.

**YIELD: 15 PIECES**

# Chocolate Cupcakes

*Wheat- and dairy-free.*

| | |
|---|---|
| 1 | cup maple crystals or date sugar |
| 3/4 | cup whole spelt flour |
| 3/4 | cup cocoa powder |
| 1/2 | cup unbleached white spelt flour |
| 1 1/2 | teaspoons baking soda |
| 1 | teaspoon baking powder |
| 1 | cup water |
| 3/4 | cup extra-virgin olive oil |
| 1/2 | cup unsweetened applesauce |
| 2 | tablespoons apple cider vinegar |
| 1 | teaspoon vanilla extract |
| | Pinch of sea salt |

1. Preheat oven to 325°F.

2. Place paper liners in two 12-cup muffin pans.

3. Sift the maple crystals or date sugar, whole spelt flour, cocoa, white spelt flour, baking soda, and baking powder together into a large mixing bowl, and stir several times with a large wooden spoon to combine.

4. Place the water, oil, applesauce, vinegar, vanilla, and salt in a blender and blend until smooth and well combined, about 30 seconds.

5. Fold the wet ingredients into the dry ingredients and stir several times until well combined. Do not leave any lumps. Fill each prepared baking cup ¾ full with batter.

6. Bake for 15 to 20 minutes, or until a toothpick inserted in the middle of a cupcake pulls out cleanly. Let cupcakes cool before removing them from the pan. Allow them to cool completely before icing.

**YIELD: 24 CUPCAKES**

# Chocolate Tofu Whip

*Use as a frosting for cupcakes or as a mousse dessert with chopped strawberries.*

| | |
|---|---|
| 1 | package (16 ounces) silken tofu |
| 1³/₄ | cups (10 ounces) chocolate chips (preferably barley sweetened, like Sunspire) |
| 3 | tablespoons maple syrup |
| 1 | teaspoon vanilla extract |
| | Pinch of sea salt |

1. Line a sieve with paper towels and place the tofu inside. Pull up the paper towels to cover the tofu, and weight with a can laid on its side or two or three stacked bowls. Allow the tofu to drain for 15 minutes, or until about ⅓ cup of the liquid has drained out.

2. Blend the tofu in a food processor or blender just until smooth.

3. In a double boiler, soften the chocolate chips with the maple syrup over low heat. Stir gently with a rubber spatula until melted and combined.

4. Add the chocolate mixture with vanilla and salt to the tofu in the food processor or blender. Add the vanilla and salt and mix until creamy, scraping down sides once or twice to ensure complete incorporation.

5. Scrape the tofu whip into an airtight glass container and refrigerate for 1 hour or until set.

**YIELD: 3 CUPS**

# COCONUT DATE ROLLS

   2    **cups fresh dates, pitted (preferably Medjool dates)**

   1    **cup unsweetened shredded coconut**

1. Pulse the dates in a food processor fitted with a normal blade 15 to 20 times.

2. Move the pulverized dates to a mixing bowl and stir in the coconut with a wooden spoon.

3. Spoon out 2 tablespoons at a time and roll into log shapes with your hands.

4. Store in an airtight container in the refrigerator for up to a week.

5. Serve cold or at room temperature.

**YIELD: 20 ROLLS**

# CRUNCHY CRANBERRIES, APPLES, AND PEARS

   1    **Granny Smith apple, halved and cored**

   1    **firm pear, halved and cored**

   1    **tablespoon lemon juice**

   3    **tablespoons fresh or frozen cranberries**

   2    **fresh Medjool dates, pitted and quartered**

  1/4    **cup pecans, coarsely chopped**

  1 1/2    **teaspoons powdered cinnamon**

  1/4    **teaspoon freshly grated nutmeg**

   1    **teaspoon real vanilla extract**

  1/4    **cup brown rice syrup**

1. Preheat oven to 325°F.

2. Rub the cut apple and pear with the lemon juice to stop them from turning brown.

3. Cut a small slice off of the rounded side of each fruit half, so that they lay flat without tipping over.

4. Place the apple and pear halves with the cut sides facing up and fill each core with the cranberries and dates.

5. Mix the pecans, cinnamon, nutmeg, vanilla, and rice syrupto-gether in a bowl and spread the mixture evenly over the fruit.

6. Bake for 30 minutes.

**YIELD: 4 HALVES**


# Maple Pecan Cookies

*Wheat-free and naturally sweetened.*

| | |
|---|---|
| 2½ | cups pecans, ground in food processor until size of small pebbles |
| 2 | cups quick oats, ground |
| 1 | cup unbleached white spelt flour, sifted |
| 1 | cup whole spelt flour, sifted |
| 1 | cup maple syrup |
| ½ | cup unrefined coconut oil |
| 1 | tablespoon real vanilla extract |
| ¼ | teaspoon sea salt |
| 15 | pecan halves |

1. Preheat oven to 350°F.

2. Line a baking sheet with parchment paper.

3. In a large mixing bowl, combine the ground pecans, oats, and sifted white spelt and whole spelt flours.

4. In a medium mixing bowl, whisk together the maple syrup, oil, vanilla, and sea salt.

5. Mix the wet ingredients into the dry and stir well to combine.

6. Scoop ¼ cup of dough onto lined baking sheet and gently press down using your palm. Repeat with remaining dough. Press a pecan half into the top of each cookie.

7. Bake for 12 to 14 minutes or until golden brown.

**YIELD: 30 COOKIES**

# Nutty Rice Bars

   $\frac{1}{2}$   cup natural nut butter (peanut, pecan, almond, or cashew are great)

   $\frac{1}{2}$   cup brown rice syrup or agave nectar

   3   cups unsweetened puffed rice cereal

   $\frac{1}{4}$   cup coarsely chopped nuts

1. Lightly oil an 8" × 8" glass baking dish and a large mixing bowl, using extra-virgin olive oil or melted coconut oil.

2. In a small saucepan, combine the nut butter and syrup or nectar. Place over low heat and stir carefully until mixture is melted and completely blended. Remove from heat.

3. Lightly oil your hands. In the large oiled mixing bowl, mix the cereal and nuts together with the nut butter mixture.

4. Press the mixture into the baking dish and cover with plastic wrap. Refrigerate for 1 hour or until firm. Cut into 2-inch squares and serve.

**YIELD: 16 2" BARS**

# OATMEAL RAISIN COOKIES

*Wheat- and dairy-free.*

| | |
|---|---|
| 1 | cup whole spelt flour |
| $3/4$ | cup rolled oats |
| $3/4$ | cup quick oats |
| $1/4$ | teaspoon sea salt |
| $1/4$ | teaspoon baking powder |
| $1/4$ | teaspoon baking soda |
| $1/4$ | teaspoon cinnamon |
| $1/8$ | teaspoon fresh nutmeg |
| $1/2$ | cup maple syrup |
| $1/4$ | cup + 2 tablespoons unrefined coconut oil or extra-virgin olive oil |
| 3 | tablespoons rice, soy, or almond milk |
| $1/4$ | teaspoon apple cider vinegar |
| $3/4$ | cup raisins |

1. Preheat oven to 350°F.

2. Line a cookie sheet with parchment paper and set aside.

3. Sift the spelt flour into a large mixing bowl and add the rolled oats, quick oats, salt, baking powder, baking soda, cinnamon, and nutmeg. Stir well to combine.

4. In a medium mixing bowl, combine the maple syrup, oil, milk, and vinegar. Whisk well and pour the wet ingredients into the dry.

5. Add the raisins and stir with a large wooden spoon or rubber spatula until the raisins are mixed in.

6. Drop about 2 tablespoons of batter per cookie onto the lined baking sheet.

7. Bake for 13 to 15 minutes or until golden brown.

**YIELD: 11 COOKIES**

# Raw Chocolate Pudding

- 10    fresh dates, pitted and cut in quarters
- 10    dried figs, stems removed, cut in quarters
- 2    tablespoons unsweetened cocoa powder
- 2    tablespoons raw nut butter (optional)
- 1    teaspoon vanilla extract
- 1½–2    cups filtered water

1. Place the dates, figs, cocoa, nut butter (if using), vanilla, and 1 cup of water in a blender and pulse several times until the fruits begin to break down.
2. Blend until smooth and creamy, slowly adding water as needed for desired consistency.

**YIELD: 2½ CUPS**


# Sweet and Beany Popsicles

- 2    cups cooked, drained, and cooled white cannellini beans, unsalted
- 1    cup almond milk or vanilla flavored soy or rice milk
- 1    teaspoon cinnamon
- 1    large ripe banana
- 3    tablespoons maple syrup
- 1½    teaspoons real vanilla extract

1. Place the beans, milk, cinnamon, banana, maple syrup, and vanilla in a blender and blend well until smooth and creamy. Add more milk for a more pourable mix.
2. Pour the mix into popsicle molds or ice cube trays and add clean popsicle sticks or toothpicks for handles.
3. Freeze for at least 3 hours for firm popsicles.

**YIELD: 10 3-OUNCE POPSICLES**

# Vanilla Tofu Cream

*Use as a dip for fruit or as an icing spread for scones or cakes.*

- 1 package (16 ounces) silken tofu
- 3/4 cup unsweetened nut butter (almond, peanut, etc.)
- 4 tablespoons maple syrup or brown rice syrup
- 1 tablespoon pure vanilla extract

  Pinch of sea salt

1. Line a sieve with paper towels and place the tofu inside. Pull up the paper towels to cover the tofu, and weight with a can laid on its side or two or three stacked bowls. Allow tofu to drain for 15 minutes, or until about 1/3 cup of the liquid has drained out.

2. Place the drained tofu, nut butter, syrup, vanilla, and salt in a food processor fitted with a blade. Process until smooth, scraping down the sides of the bowl once or twice.

3. To set up, or harden slightly, refrigerate the cream for 2 hours.

4. Refrigerate in an airtight container for up to 5 days.

**YIELD: 2 CUPS**

# Whole Vanilla Cake

*Work gently with this cake as it is a bit more delicate than cakes not made with whole flour. Use unsweetened fruit spread or hardened chocolate tofu spread or Vanilla Tofu Cream (see page 267) as icing.*

| | |
|---|---|
| 1 | tablespoon (for dusting cake pan) + 2¼ cups whole spelt flour |
| 3 | teaspoons baking powder |
| | Pinch of sea salt |
| ⅓ | cup mild vegetable oil or coconut oil |
| ½ | cup maple syrup |
| 1 | teaspoon grated lemon zest |
| 2 | teaspoons pure vanilla extract |
| 1 | cup soy, almond, or rice milk |

1. Preheat oven to 350°F.

2. Lightly oil a 9-inch cake pan and dust with 1 tablespoon of the flour, turning the pan to evenly coat the entire bottom and edges with flour.

3. In a large mixing bowl, sift together the remaining flour, baking powder, and salt.

4. In a medium mixing bowl, whisk together the oil, maple syrup, lemon zest, vanilla, and milk until completely combined and smooth.

5. Gently stir the wet ingredients into the flour, mixing until just smooth. Do not overmix, which will cause the cake to be tough. The batter should not be runny.

6. Scrape the batter into the prepared pan and bake on the center rack in the oven for 40 minutes, or until a toothpick inserted in the middle comes out clean.

7. Allow cake to cool for 10 minutes before delicately removing from pan.

**YIELD: 1 9″ CAKE**

# Products for Transitioning

## CAFFEINE

### HERBAL COFFEE

Teeccino
Flavors of herbal coffee include Vanilla Nut, Hazelnut, Almond Amaretto, Original, Java, Mocha, and Chocolate Mint
800-498-3434
www.teeccino.com

### TEA

Celestial Seasonings
Roastaroma herb tea
800-351-8175
www.celestialseasonings.com

Yogi Tea
Varieties of exotic tea include DeCaffé Roast, Vanilla Hazelnut, and Cocoa Spice Teas
800-964-4832
www.yogitea.com

## CARBOHYDRATES

### BAKING MIXES

Arrowhead Mills
Gluten-free pancake and baking mixes, sugar-free puffed grain cereals, and whole grains
800-434-4246
www.arrowheadmills.com

Bob's Red Mill
Whole grains and gluten-free baking mixes and flours
800-349-2173
www.bobsredmill.com

Sylvan Border Farms
Gluten-free baking mixes
800-297-5399
www.sylvanborderfarm.com

## BREADS

Mana
Frozen wheat- and yeast-free
   breads
866-972-6879
www.naturespath.com

## CEREALS

*Barbara's
Naturally sweetened boxed
   cereals
707-765-2273
www.barbarasbakery.com

Nature's Path
Sugar-free puffed grain
   cereals
866-972-6879
www.naturespath.com

## PASTAS

Eden
Wheat-free mung bean
   pastas
888-441-3336
www.edenfoods.com

Tinkyada
Gluten- and wheat-free
   pastas
416-609-0016
www.tinkyada.com

Vita Spelt
Wheat-free pastas
517-351-9231
www.purityfoods.com

# DAIRY ALTERNATIVES

## MARGARINE

Earth Balance
Nonhydrogenated vegetable
   margarine
201-568-9300
www.earthbalance.net

## MILK

Edensoy
Organic plain, vanilla, and
   chocolate-flavored soy
   milks
888-441-3336
www.edenfoods.com

*Pacific
Soy and oat milks
503-692-9666
www.pacificfoods.com

Rice Dream
Plain, vanilla, and chocolate-
   flavored rice milks
800-434-4246
www.imaginefoods.com

# FAT

## COOKING OILS (ORGANIC)

Bionaturae
860-642-6996
www.bionaturae.com/
   contact.html

Spectrum Naturals
866-972-6879
www.spectrumorganics.com

## NUT BUTTERS

Maranatha
Natural nut butters
888-441-3336
www.nspiredfoods.com/
maranatha.html

Once Again Nut Butter
Natural nut butters free of
sugar and hydrogenated fats
888-800-8075
www.onceagainnutbutter.com

# PROTEIN

## BEANS

Arrowhead Mills
Organic dried beans
800-434-4246
www.arrowheadmills.com

Bob's Red Mill
Organic dried beans
800-349-2173
www.bobsredmill.com

Eden
Organic canned beans
888-441-3336
www.edenfoods.com

Westbrae Natural
Organic canned beans
800-434-4246
www.westbrae.com

## MEATLESS "MEAT" PRODUCTS

*Lightlife
Meatless tofu hot dogs, fake
bacon, and lunch meats
800-SOY-EASY (769-3279)
www.lightlife.com

*Yves
Meatless sausages and lunch
meats
800-667-9837
www.yvesveggie.com

# SEA VEGETABLES

Eden
888-441-3336
www.edenfoods.com

Main Coast Sea Vegetables
207-565-2907
www.seaveg.com

# SUGAR

## AGAVE NECTAR

Sweet Cactus Farms
310-733-4343
www.sweetcactusfarms.com

## BARLEY MALT

Eden
888-441-3336
www.edenfoods.com

## BROWN RICE SYRUP

Lundberg
530-882-4551
www.lundberg.com

## DATE SUGAR

Bob's Red Mill
800-349-2173
www.bobsredmill.com

## GRAIN-SWEETENED CHOCOLATE CHIPS AND UNSWEETENED CAROB CHIPS

Sunspire
510-686-0116
www.nspiredfoods.com

## STEVIA LIQUIDS AND POWDERS

Stevia Smart
www.steviasmart.com

**\*REMEMBER:** Be a good food detective! Some products contain added natural sugars, so always read labels.

# A Week's Worth of Sample Detox Menus

## MONDAY

**BREAKFAST:**   *Hearty Morning Oatmeal Porridge (page 180)*

**LUNCH:**   *Falafel Chickpea Patties (page 251)*

*Easy Bein' Green Sauté (page 250)*

**DINNER:**   *Italian-Style Beans and Greens (page 212)*

*Overnight Slaw (page 254)*

*Black Bean and Sweet Potato Chili (page 208)*

**SNACK:**   *Berry Fudgy-Cicles (page 258)*

## TUESDAY

**BREAKFAST:**   *Power Morning Shake (page 182)*

**LUNCH:**   *"Creamy" Carrot Soup (page 188)*

*Steamed greens with Easy Chutney (page 240)*

**DINNER:**   *Broccoli and Miso Calzones (page 210)*

**SNACK:**   *Nutty Rice Bars (page 264)*

## WEDNESDAY

**BREAKFAST:** *Orange Date Scones (page 181)*

**LUNCH:** *Italian-Style Crispy Cauliflower (page 252) with Gomasio (page 241)*

*Milanese Tomato Soup (page 189)*

**DINNER:** *Mushroom Barley Pilaf (page 231)*

*Simple green salad with Lemony Garlic Mustard Salad Dressing (page 244)*

**DESSERT:** *Maple Pecan Cookies (page 263)*

## THURSDAY

**BREAKFAST:** *Carrot Muffins (page 227)*

*Almond Milk (page 184)*

**LUNCH:** *Miso Stew (page 194)*

**DINNER:** *Guacamole (page 242) and carrot sticks, bell pepper slices, and celery sticks*

*Corn and Kidney Bean Chili (page 209)*

*Polenta (page 232)*

**SNACK:** *Savory Seeds (page 246) and Watermelon Cooler (page 188)*

## FRIDAY

**BREAKFAST:** *Wheat-Free Pancakes with Blueberry Syrup (page 183) and Homemade Nut Butter (page 243)*

**LUNCH:** *Sang Choy Bow (Chinese Mushroom Rice "Burritos") (page 216)*

**DINNER:** *Savory Stuffed Acorn Squash (page 217)*

*Baked Tempeh (page 207)*

*Corny Corn Bread (page 229)*

*Cranberry Relish (page 238)*

**DESSERT:** *Crunchy Cranberries, Apples, and Pears (page 262)*

## SATURDAY

**BREAKFAST:**   *Breakfast Patties (page 178)*

*Sassy Homemade Applesauce (page 246)*

**LUNCH:**   *Parsley, Sage, Rosemary, and Thyme Rice (page 232)*

*Nori Wrap-Ups (page 253)*

**DINNER:**   *Popeye's Spinach Pie (page 214)*

*Refreshing and Cleansing Radish Salad (page 202)*

*Raw Chocolate Pudding (page 266)*

## SUNDAY

**BREAKFAST:**   *Breakfast Tofu Scramble for One (page 179)*

*Sunny Citrus Tea (page 185)*

**LUNCH:**   *Neptune's Noodle Soup (page 196)*

*Steamed broccoli with Curry Dressing (page 238)*

**DINNER:**   *Walnut Burger Patties (page 225) with Sun-Dried Tomato Spread (page 247)*

*Spicy Sweet Potato Fries (page 255)*

*Ketchup (page 244)*

# Diet Diversity: Why Different Cultures Eat Different Things

**Why do some cultures eat** diets rich in fish while others eat only the protein found in wild game? Why do some build a diet around rice while others build their diet around potatoes? It's all about the earth and what she provides in any given location.

There is a strong link between where we came from, in the evolutionary sense, and what foods are helpful to us. Would you ask a hunter-gatherer from the Amazon rain forest to eat a diet of olive oil, pasta, and wine? Not only would it be impossible for our jungle-dweller to find such foods, but perhaps his body runs better when he eats the traditional diet of that region, which includes fruits, vegetables, and fish that are plentiful where he lives.

Our bodies have evolved naturally to enable us to eat and process those foods that are most readily available to us. The diversity of world diets is testament to how truly unique and individual we all are. Take a look at these world diet overviews. You may learn a thing or two about your dietary heritage.

Remember, too, that it only makes sense that if we eat a diet that reflects the traditional diet of our own inherited ethnic group, we'll likely feel better.

**AFRICAN BANTU:** largely vegetarian, bananas, beans, corn, insects, millet, sorghum, sweet potatoes, small amounts of dairy and meat

**CANADIAN FIRST NATIONS:** berries, caribou, fish, nuts, seal, vegetables

**CARIBBEAN:** allspice, chicken, crab, fish, garlic, ginger, greens, limes, okra, pork, rice, spicy peppers, yams

**CHINESE:** a minimum of animal meats for most of the population, beans, cabbage, eggs, fermented pickles, fermented soy products, greens, honey, leek, onion, plums, radishes, small amounts of rice syrup, scallions, sweet potatoes, whole grains (rice, wheat, millet)

**EASTERN EUROPEAN:** beets and beet greens, cabbages, fish, game, kasha or buckwheat

**EGYPTIAN:** almonds, beans, berries, birds, cabbages, chickpeas, coriander, cucumbers, endive, figs, fish, garlic, grapes, melons, olives, onions, peaches, pomegranates, radishes, raisins, whole wheat bread

**GERMAN:** beef, beer, cabbage, eggs, game, greens, kale, lentils, mushrooms, mustard, naturally fermented sauerkraut, onion, pork, rabbit, sausages, trout, whole rye breads

**HAWAIIAN/POLYNESIAN:** fish; high-fiber, complex carbs; pineapple; poi; sea vegetables; sweet potatoes; taro root

**IRANIAN:** asparagus, barley, basil, broad beans, cheese, chestnuts, chicken, chickpeas, cows, cucumbers, dates, fish, garden cress, garlic, goats, grapes, lentils, melons, millet, onions, plums, pomegranates, quince, radishes, rice, saffron, spinach, walnuts, wheat, yogurt

**IRISH AND BRITISH ISLES:** beef; duck; egg; fish; lamb; mushrooms; onions; organ meats; pickled vegetables; pork; rabbit; root vegetables; sea vegetables; whole dairy milk and butter; whole rye, barley, and oats

**JAPANESE:** fermented soy foods, fish, fruit, green leafy vegetables, radishes, rice, sea vegetables, small amounts of meat and pork

**JEWISH:** almonds, apples, barley, beans, cabbage, chestnuts, chicken, chickpeas, eggplant, eggs, figs, herring, honey, matzo, meat, mushrooms, olives and olive oil, onions, peppers, pomegranates, poppy seeds, potatoes, raisins, sweet potatoes, wheat

**MAASAI AND OTHER MEAT HERDERS:** acacia, cow's blood and meat, fruits and vegetables, milk, myrrh, small amounts of fish, whole grains as sour or fermented porridges

**MEDITERRANEAN:** sparing use of meat and eggs, chickpeas, fish, garlic, grapes and other fruit, herbs, legumes, nuts, olive oil, seeds, vegetables and greens, whole grain breads and pastas

**MEXICAN:** amaranth, avocados, beans, cabbage, chile peppers, cilantro, coconut, corn, fish, green vegetables, papayas, peanuts, pineapples, radishes, squash, sweet potatoes, tomatoes, small amounts of meats including ducks, pigeons, turkey, and venison

**NATIVE AMERICAN:** animal foods of every description, with a heavy emphasis on organ meats, the higher in fat the better; agave, beans, berries, corn, fish, maple, nuts, pumpkins, wild greens, wild rice

**RUSSIAN:** beef; beets; cabbage, fish; game; millet; mushrooms; nuts; onion; turnips; whole rye, wheat, or oat breads

**SCANDINAVIAN:** apples, beets, berries, cabbage, cucumbers, dill, fish, herring, horseradish, mushrooms, mussels, nuts, oysters, parsley, pork, poultry, reindeer, rye, salmon

**SOUTH AMERICAN:** small amounts of red meats, beans, chicken, eggs, fish, fruits, legumes, nuts, potatoes, tubers, vegetables, whole grain quinoa

**SPANISH:** almonds, chicken, cinnamon, fish, garlic, ham, nuts, olives, peppers, pork, saffron, sesame, shellfish

**THAI:** bananas, black and mung beans, cabbage, coconut meat and oil, eggplant, fish, fresh herbs and spices, onions, plums, rice, tamarind

**WESTERN NILE/SUDAN:** fish, green vegetables, lentils, peanuts, whole grains

It is interesting to note that modern disease rates among some of these cultures are linked directly to their diets being modified as the American diet has been, by the addition of refined flours, sugars, and processed foods. So although some cultures traditionally ate diets that were, say, high in animal protein, this was (and would still be) a balanced, healthy approach for people indigenous to that environment.

# Pantry Staples: The Essential Foods and Spices to Have in Your Kitchen

**APPLE CIDER VINEGAR:** Find an organic and unfiltered or unpasteurized variety. The traditionally made variety is free of chemicals and preservatives. Has been used as a tonic for circulation and balancing the body's acidity, and has a high potassium content. Great for dressings, condiments, and marinades.

**BALSAMIC VINEGAR:** The best of these delicious Italian vinegars are labeled "traditionally brewed" or "traditionally fermented."

**BROWN RICE SYRUP:** A mild, nutty sweetener, great for tea, cereals, and baking.

**DRIED BEANS:** Store in glass containers out of direct sunlight.

**DRIED FRUIT:** Store dried apple slices, banana chips, dates, mangoes, and raisins in airtight glass containers in a cool, dark place.

**DRIED MUSHROOMS:** Stored in a sealable plastic bag, dried mushrooms will keep well for several months.

**EXTRA-VIRGIN OLIVE OIL:** Look for organic, unprocessed oils in dark or opaque bottles.

**GARLIC:** Store fresh heads in a dark, cool drawer. Do not store in the refrigerator. Should keep for several months.

**GINGER:** Fresh ginger can be stored in the refrigerator door, and dried ginger can be stored on your spice rack.

**GOMASIO:** A tasty traditional Japanese condiment of lightly toasted sesame seeds and sea salt. Use instead of straight salt to flavor your food. High in calcium, iron, and vitamins A and B.

**HERBS AND SPICES:** Basil, black pepper, cayenne, chili powder, cinnamon, curry powder, marjoram, parsley, rosemary, sage, thyme, and turmeric. Store away from heat and direct sunlight. Do not store next to the stove or on top of the refrigerator.

**HOT SAUCE:** Adds some kick to simple vegetables, soups, beans, and grains. Look for a hot sauce without added sugar or preservatives.

**MAPLE SYRUP:** Grade B is the darker, more flavorful variety.

**NATURALLY BREWED SOY SAUCE (TAMARI, SHOYU, OR BRAGG'S LIQUID AMINOS):** Has less sodium than an equal amount of salt and is a great flavor enhancer. Commercially made soy sauces are produced with a variety of chemicals and have a sharper, bitter taste.

**ONIONS:** Hang onions in a cool, well-ventilated place. Do not refrigerate.

**RICE CAKES:** Come in a variety of flavors with other grains, sea vegetables, and added spices. Look for unsweetened varieties in health food stores.

**SEA SALT:** Offering a richer taste than refined, iodized salt, unrefined sea salts often look gray and damp. This look is because of the rich mineral content of the salt.

**SEA VEGETABLES:** Stored in a sealable plastic bag, sea vegetables keep well for a year or more. Great for soups and bean dishes.

**SEEDS (POPPY, PUMPKIN, SESAME, AND SUNFLOWER):** Wonderful for sprinkling on top of dishes, seeds provide a crunchy texture, extra protein, and healthy fats. Hulled seeds require refrigeration.

**SESAME OIL:** The toasted variety provides more flavor than the original version.

**TAHINI:** Also known as sesame butter, tahini is great for creamy sauces and adds protein and healthy fat.

**TOMATO SAUCE:** Canned varieties of diced, whole, and pureed tomatoes are versatile and common in recipes.

**UME VINEGAR:** A traditional Japanese seasoning liquid, and technically not a vinegar, umeboshi vinegar can be used to replace salt and vinegar in recipes.

**UNREFINED COCONUT OIL:** Use organic, unprocessed oil for the best quality.

**WHOLE GRAINS:** Store in glass containers in a cool, dark place or in the refrigerator. The natural oils in grains may begin to degrade after a while.

# Web Sites You'll Like

www.edenfoods.com

www.garynull.com

www.goya.com

www.healthychefalex.com

www.kitchengardeners.org

www.mercola.com

www.mindfully.org

www.naturalfiberclothing.com

www.naturalgourmetschool.com

www.optimalhealthconcepts.com

www.organicconsumers.org

www.rachel.org

www.rapunzel.com

www.vegweb.com

# Additional Reading

A Short History of Nearly Everything by Bill Bryson

Ayurveda: The Ancient Indian Science of Healing by Ashok Majumdar

Ayurveda for Health and Well-Being by Shanti Gowans

Better Basics for the Home by Annie-Berthold Bond

Creating Health: Beyond Prevention, toward Perfection by Deepak Chopra

Creating Wholeness: A Self-Healing Workbook Using Dynamic Relaxation, Images, and Thoughts by Erik Peper and Catherine F. Holt

Don't Eat This Book: Fast Food and the Supersizing of America by Morgan Spurlock

The Energy Balance Diet by Joshua Rosenthal

Fast Food Nation by Eric Schlosser

Food and Our Bones by Annemarie Colbin

Foods That Fight Pain by Dr. Neal Barnard

For Women Only! by Gary Null

The Gluten-Free Gourmet, Second Edition: Living Well without Wheat by Bette Hagman

If the Buddha Came to Dinner by Halé Sofia Schatz

Prescription for Dietary Wellness by Phyllis A. Balch, CNC

The Real Cause of Heart Disease Is Not Cholesterol by Paul A. Stitt

The Vegetarian Handbook by Gary Null

The New Whole Foods Encyclopedia by Rebecca Wood

You Can Heal Your Life by Louise L. Hay

# Organizations That Support the Detox Lifestyle

**Institute for Integrative Nutrition**
120 West 41st Street, 2nd Floor
New York, NY 10036
212-730-5433
www.integrativenutrition.com

**Kitchen Gardeners International**
7 Flintlock Drive
Scarborough, ME 04074
207-883-1107
www.kitchengardeners.org

**Mind-Body Medical Institute**
824 Boylston Street
Chestnut Hill, MA 02467
866-509-0732
www.mbmi.org

**The Natural Gourmet Cookery School**
48 West 21st Street, 2nd Floor
New York, NY 10010
212-645-5170
www.naturalgourmetschool.com

**Natural Ovens Bakery**
4300 County Highway CR
Manitowoc, WI 54220
800-558-3535
www.naturalovens.com

**The Weston A. Price Foundation**
PMB 106–380
4200 Wisconsin Avenue NW
Washington, DC 20016
202-333-HEAL (4325)
www.westonaprice.org

# Index

Underscored page references indicate boxed text and tables.

# C

Cabbage
  Overnight Slaw, 254
Caffeine
  addiction to, 41–42, 87–88
  children consuming, 91–92
  detoxing from, 92–94
  health effects of, 84–86, 88–90
  history of, 86–87
  sleep problems from, 90
  water consumption with, 54–55
Cake
  Chocolate Cupcakes, 260
  Whole Vanilla Cake, 268
Calcium
  daily requirements for, 139
  loss of, from milk drinking, 134–35
  nondairy sources of, 139, <u>140</u>
Calzones
  Broccoli and Miso Calzones,
    210–11
*Candida albicans* bacteria, in colon,
  31, 32, 76–77
Candles, avoiding air pollution
  from, 153–54
Carbohydrates
  allergies to, 118–20
  assesssing reaction to, <u>116</u>
  complex, 65
    fiber in, 115–16
    in whole grains, 43, 74, 114,
      120–21 (*see also* Whole
      grains)
  as energy source, 42, 65
  glycemic index of, 116–17
  refined, 42–43, 64–65, 74
  understanding labeling on, 117–18
Carpet, indoor air pollution from,
  153
Carrots
  Carrot Muffins, 227
  "Creamy" Carrot Soup, 190
  Roasted Veggies and Savory
    Quinoa Salad, 203
  Veggie Pâté, 256
Cauliflower
  Italian-Style Crispy Cauliflower,
    252

Celiac disease, 118–19, 121
Cells, role of, 30
Cheese consumption, 137
Chickpeas
  Chickpea Lemon Spinach Salad,
    199
  Falafel Chickpea Patties, 251
Chili
  Black Bean and Sweet Potato
    Chili, 208
  Corn and Kidney Bean Chili, 209
Chocolate
  Chocolate Anthills, 259
  Chocolate Cupcakes, 260
  Chocolate Tofu Whip, 261
  Raw Chocolate Pudding, 266
Chutney
  Easy Chutney, 240–41
Cleaning products, household
  natural, 152, 154–55, <u>155</u>
  toxins in, 150–52
Clothing, toxins in, 156
Clutter, eliminating, 157
Coconut
  Coconut Curry Rice, 228
  Coconut Date Rolls, 262
Coffee. *See also* Caffeine
  decaffeinated, switching to, 93
  health effects of, 89–90
  history of, 86–87
Colon
  bacterial overgrowth in, 31–32,
    76–77
  cleansing, 166
Constipation, 166
Cookies
  Maple Pecan Cookies, 263
  Oatmeal Raisin Cookies, 265
Cooking, with music, 82
Corn
  Corn, Mushroom, and Potato
    Chowder, 189
  Corn and Kidney Bean Chili, 209
  Corny Corn Bread, 229
Corn allergy, 120
Cornmeal
  Corny Corn Bread, 229
  Polenta, 232–33

Food safety issues, 137–38

Fruits. *See also specific fruits*

## G

Ganjhu, Lisa, on preventive eating, x–xii

Glycemic index, 116–17

Goal-setting, 168

Gomasio, 241

Grains. *See* Whole grains; *specific grains*

Grain sensitivities, 121–24

Granola

  Apple Granola Muffins, 176–77

Greens

  Asparagus, Bok Choy, and Tofu Stir-Fry, 206

  Easy Bein' Green Sauté, 250

  Italian-Style Beans and Greens, 212

  Warm Potato and Kale Salad, 205

Guacamole, 242

## H

Herbal steam bath, 165

Herbal teas, 142, 144

Herbs

  Creamy Tomato Millet with Fresh Herbs, 230

  Dill Tofu Dip, 239

  Herbed Garden Salad, 200

  Herbed Quinoa Salad, 201

  Parsley, Sage, Rosemary, and Thyme Rice, 232

High fructose corn syrup (HFCS), 65–66, 67

High-protein diets, health problems from, 128–29, 130–31

Home environment

  air pollution in, 152–54

  detoxifying, 145–46, 148, 149, 149, 152, 153–55, 156

  natural cleaning products for, 152, 154–55, 155

  sources of toxins in

    beauty products, 155–56

    clothing, 156

    household cleaning products, 150–52

plastics, 146–48, 149

pots and pans, 149

Hot skin scrub, 166–67

Household cleaning products

  natural, 152, 154–55, 155

  toxins in, 150–52

Hydrogenated fat. *See* Trans fat

## I

Indoor air pollution, 152–54

Insulin resistance, 68–69

## J

Jam

  Red Raspberry Jam, 245

Jamieson, Alex

  childhood lifestyle of, 3–5, 8

  culinary and nutritional training of, 10–12

  Detox Diet designed by, viii, 20–23, 35, 36, 37, 40

  diet mistakes of, 5–7

  Dr. Ganjhu on, x–xi

  personal detox experience of, 7–9

  *Super Size Me* and, vii–viii, 13–23

Junk food, eliminating, 60–61

## K

Kale

  Easy Bein' Green Sauté, 250

  Italian-Style Beans and Greens, 212

  Warm Potato and Kale Salad, 205

Ketchup, 244

Kidney health, 52–53

Kitchen, detoxifying, 60–61

## L

Lactose intolerance, 135, 136, 139

Laughter, 169

Leeks

  "Creamy" Potato Leek Soup, 191

Leftovers, from recipes, 173

Lemons

  Chickpea Lemon Spinach Salad, 199

  Citrus Avocado Pesto, 237

  Lemony Garlic Mustard Salad Dressing, 244

  Safely Sweet Lemonade, 185

Lentils
  Veggie Pâté, 256
  Walnut Lentil Salad, 204
Lettuce
  Nori or Lettuce Leaf Wrap-Ups,
    253
Liver
  effect of trans fat on, 101, 102
  foods supporting, <u>103</u>
Loaf
  Veggie Loaf, 224

# M

Massage, 167
McDonald's
  additives used by, 29–30
  cost control of, 28
  nutritional claims of, vii, 13, 19,
    24
  nutritional information on, 20,
    <u>20–21</u>
  in *Super Size Me*, 14, 16, 17, 18
  trans fat and, 100
Meat, 37, 40, 133–34
Meditation, 167–68
Meditative breathing, 164–65
Mental detox techniques
  analzying causes of stress, 96
  body appreciation, 112
  communing with nature, 157–58
  creating detox road map, 62–63
  mind-body connection, 169–70
  releasing fears, 144
  researching origin of foods,
    126–27
  understanding source of sugar
    addiction, 83
Menus, sample detox, 273–75
Metabolism, 30
Milk
  Almond Milk, 184
  problems related to, 134–37
  substitutions for, 141
Millet
  Creamy Tomato Millet with
    Fresh Herbs, 230
Mind-body connection, 169–70
Mindless eating, 160–62

Miso
  Broccoli and Miso Calzones,
    210–11
  Homemade Miso Tofu Cheese
    Spread, 242
  Miso Stew, 194–95
Movies about food, 126
Muffins
  Apple Granola Muffins, 176–77
  Carrot Muffins, 227
Mushrooms
  Corn, Mushroom, and Potato
    Chowder, 189
  Mushroom Barley Pilaf, 231
  Sang Choy Bow (Chinese Mush-
    room Rice "Burritos"), 216

# N

Natural sweeteners, 79–82, <u>80–81</u>
Nature, healing power of, 157–58
Noodles
  Avocado Sesame Pasta, 226
  Neptune's Noodle Soup, 196–97
  Thai Protein Noodle Salad, 218–19
  Vietnamese Noodle Soup, 198
Nori
  Nori or Lettuce Leaf Wrap-Ups,
    253
Nut butter
  Homemade Nut Butter, 243
  Nutty Rice Bars, 264
Nuts. *See also specific nuts*
  essential fatty acids in, 105–6
  storing, 106

# O

Oatmeal
  Hearty Morning Oatmeal
    Porridge, 180
  Oatmeal Raisin Cookies, 265
  sweetened, in packets, 14
Obesity, effects of, 33
Oils
  as butter replacement, 141
  for cooking, 107, 109–10
  with essential fatty acids, 105
  manufacture and extraction of,
    106–7

# Acknowledgments

This book was inspired by the hundreds of writers, teachers, and healers whose work has had an impact on my life. I would like to thank my Rodale editor, Margot Schupf; angel and daily editor Emily Heckman; my fantastic agent, Elyse Cheney; Dr. Lisa Ganjhu; Dr. Neal Barnard; and Taffy Elrod, my wonderful chef-friend who tested all these recipes and offered me a kind ear and tasty rice pudding whenever I needed it. I would also like to thank Annemarie Colbin for founding the Natural Gourmet Cookery School and Joshua Rosenthal for founding the Institute for Integrative Nutrition. Both of these schools helped me on the path to healthy living and instructed me on how to make a living while doing something I believe in. A special thanks to all my clients, who have inspired me and helped me to learn more, and who work so hard to change their health and their lives for the better. To my friends and family, who have always supported me, loved me, and offered me real nourishment. Thanks to Mom, Dad, and Eileen; Brendan Jamieson; Brendan Goodnaugh; Bridget Jamieson; Morgan; Bushka; Bo; Paul and Sean; Mimi; Ric; Kelly; Rob; Christoph; Geoffrey; Zachary; Mike; Elisabeth; Sean; Courtney; Susan and Roisin; Ana Homayoun; Amy Madden; Jeremy Chilnick; and Bob Wallace—I love you all.